CURES

11-25-82

Maybe this can
help for whatever
ails ya!

Love

Dutcher

CURES

Written by Terry Clifford

Designed by Sam Antupit

Illustrated by chas b slackman

MACMILLAN PUBLISHING CO., INC.
NEW YORK

Macmillan Publishing Co., Inc.
866 Third Avenue, New York, N.Y. 10022
Collier Macmillan Canada, Ltd.

Library of Congress Cataloging in Publication Data
Clifford, Terry.
　Cures.

　Bibliography: p.
　Includes index.
　1. Therapeutics—Popular works.　2. Materia
medica, Vegetable.　3. Folk medicine.　I. Title.
RM122.5.C54　　615.5　　80-21232
ISBN 0-02-526200-9

10 9 8 7 6 5 4 3 2 1

Printed in the United States of America

CONTENTS

Note to the Reader .... *vi*

Introduction .... *vii*

Cures *2*

Appendixes
*General Directions for Taking
the Cures* *133*

The Holistic Health Diet *139*

Selected Sources *141*

Index *143*

NOTE TO THE READER

The "cures" contained in this book are not meant to replace necessary professional medical treatment and should never be substituted for it. The author is not prescribing cures, but simply reporting their use in folk medicine and nontraditional healing systems. If you wish to use these cures in home remedies, remember that in cases of serious disease or chronic warning symptoms you should always consult a qualified physician. Even gentle herbs and nature remedies can be misused, so please consult the Appendix for additional information on dosage and application.

INTRODUCTION

Perhaps cures don't really cure at all but simply act, instead, as catalysts that enable the body to cure itself. Maybe that's what Hippocrates meant when he said, ''Natural forces within us are the true healers of disease.'' How else to explain the multitude of cures devised over the course of time, all of them claimed by their various proponents to work like magic.

From prayers to ancient medicine gods, to acupuncture and psychic healing, to remedies made from flowers and trees, to fasting, massage, water cures, and color therapy, humankind managed to heal itself with considerable success long before the advent of scientific medicine.

And while no reasonable person would dismiss the life-saving advances of modern medicine, it seems foolish to reject the healing wisdom of the past just because it is ''unscientific.'' Indeed, herbal remedies from old wives and witchdoctors provided modern science with "wonder drugs" such as digitalis, quinine, and reserpine, the first major tranquilizer.

This collection of cures from around the world serves both as a record of the lore and legend of unconventional treatments and as a practical guide to their use as home remedies (see notice on previous page). Culled from the masters and documents of different natural healing and folk medicine traditions, the cures come from widely divergent cultures and eras. What is surprising is how often disparate sources recommend the same remedy.

While the origins of the cures are dissimilar, the holistic approach from which they are derived is the same. "Holistic" is a new term for an ancient concept of healing. In the holistic view, health is largely a matter of balance and healing a matter of reconstituting it. In treating disease, therefore, holistic medicine treats the whole person and considers the forces of body, mind, and environment to be integrally related. The air we breathe, the food we eat, the way we love, the way we stand, the state of our blood, the state of our thoughts, all parts affect each other. Thus, any part may be manipulated as a means of restoring harmony to the whole.

The terms of balance vary according to different systems (the humors, elements, yin and yang energies, etc.), but the basic idea remains the same: health is a state of dynamic harmony between the inner and outer forces of nature, and each individual bears some personal responsibility for keeping this balance functional.

Natural holistic healing techniques are generally said to work more slowly but more gently than chemical drugs; they are supposed to be incorporated into a way of life that prevents disease first and cures symptoms second.

This old-fashioned approach to healing has made an unexpected comeback with the modern holistic health movement, a far-reaching phenomenon and reaction to the limits and expense of establishment medicine. Emphasizing self-care, physical fitness, and natural living, experimenting with a wide array of holistic methods—from thousand-years-old arcane remedies to modern vitamin therapy—the movement has inspired a major revival of alternative and unorthodox medicine. Folk remedies, it appears, have a remarkable capacity for enduring, as the following brief review of the basic types of holistic cures serves to point out.

NATURE CURES

Hippocrates summed up the fundamental nature cure 2,300 years ago by advising, "Let food be your medicine and medicine be your food." Nutritional medicine, particularly as a way to prevent disease, is the cornerstone of the contemporary holistic health movement, and the organic diet is its supreme panacea (see appendix for details).

Curing with nature, literally "naturopathy," is the most basic type of holistic treatment. It includes the therapeutic use of rest, fresh air, sunshine, diet, baths, massage, exercise, and medicines made from natural substances, usually sweet-smelling herbs but occasionally less endearing items such as urine.

Herbalism, the art of knowing and using the healing virtues of plants, is humanity's oldest form of clinical medicine. It has prevailed ever since medicine moved out of the realm of magic and into the sphere of applied therapeutics. Whether by observing animals (who instinctively know which grasses to eat when sick), trial and error, or the application of the "doctrine of signatures" (which holds that something about a plant's shape, color, etc., indicates its medical use), our ancestors discovered the healing qualities of plants and passed on this knowledge in written and spoken traditions.

Ancient Egyptian and Hebrew healers were herbalists, as were the physicians of classical Greece and Rome, who recorded their plant medicine teachings in books called "herbals." These works remained the standard medical references in the West throughout the Middle Ages and provided the basis for Arabic medicine as well. During the Renaissance numerous new herbals were written, the most famous being Nicholas Culpeper's in 1653. Astonishingly, it is still in print and continues to sell among modern devotees of herbal medicine.

As the natural sciences developed, herbalism declined in Europe. But if it was no longer the medicine of professional physicians, it was still the medicine of the common people. Herbal lore survived, as it always had, among itinerant herb sellers and entrenched old wives, housewives whose cookbook routinely contained recipes for remedies as well as meals. So vital were these traditions that masters of them still emerged in the twentieth century—like Maude Grieve in England and Maurice Mességué in France.

The sophisticated medical traditions of the East, notably China and India, are even older than those of the West, and have been continuously developing, it is believed, since a couple of millennia B.C. While Chinese and Indian medicine are quite different, both are highly refined systems integrally related to their native philosophies and metaphysics. Both contain huge pharmacopoeias, and their herbal remedies continue to be used by millions of people throughout Asia. Indian, Chinese, and Arabic-Greek medicine were mingled in the Tibetan medical system, and that, too, still exists today.

In North America, the folk traditions brought by the slaves from Africa, where herbal healing was a tribal art, and the settlers from the Old World combined with the medicine of the American Indians to produce a typically eclectic American result. By all accounts, the American Indians were spectacular healers who knew, among other things, the medical uses of hundreds of native plants. It is probably true that until the end of the last century a patient was better off with an Indian medicine man's herbs, sweat baths, and mystical rituals than with the blood-letting techniques of the "modern" doctors of the time.

American folk healing was practical, common knowledge, especially among blacks and rural folk, until a couple of generations ago. Prominent nature healers in America have included Benjamin Lust and Jethro Kloss.

ENERGY CURES

Another class of holistic treatment heals with the energy of nature rather than with nature itself. This subtle essence-energy is known as the "life-force" and has been identified by all mystical traditions. This life-force is said to create the energetic substratum of nature (the "subtle body"), to pervade and animate all living things, and to be, in and of itself, a healing force.

Since the life-force resides in everything natural—light, jewels, plants, and animals—one has only to tap it to release its "miraculous" healing powers. This mystical vision is not so different from Einstein's theory that solid "matter" and intangible "energy" are just different manifestations of the same thing and can be transformed into each other.

Some esoteric healing systems administer this subtle energy-essence as medicine—color healing, for example. Known to Pythagoras and various illuminati, but presently outlawed by the FDA, color therapy proceeds from the premise that energy can be divided into the seven colors of the visible spectrum, each with a specific healing quality. Gem therapy is similar, except it uses jewels, "mines of cosmic rays," to provide the needed color-energy. Aromatherapy, another subtle system, uses as medicines fragrant essential oils that work psychologically and physiologically and that are described as being like the "personality" or "spirit" of the flowers from which they're extracted (even Aristotle believed plants had "souls").

Other subtle healing systems aim at stimulating the circulation of the life-force within the human body. Such systems include: Yoga therapy (which attempts to reintegrate the body's psychophysical energies in order to promote physical health and mental peace—the longest lasting set of therapeutic exercises in the world), modern reflexology (which maintains that massage of specific spots of the feet and hands can speed the healing force to corresponding areas of the body), and Chinese acupuncture (wherein the elusive energy, understood to flow along specific but invisible pathways, is tapped and redirected by sticking pins in prescribed points all over the body—with remarkable clinical results).

MIND CURES

The medicine of magic and the supernatural, mental healing is the first and last cure, the oldest method of healing on the face of earth, and perhaps the most basic. It assigns the cause of disease to mental and spiritual factors, yet, unlike modern psychosomatic medicine, which is limited to the psychological causes of disease, it also assigns the cure of disease to the mind.

The mind medicines around today include, in part, relaxation therapy, laughter therapy, meditation, spiritual and psychic healing, hypnosis, positive thinking, biofeedback, and, of course, psychotherapy in its various forms. To some degree the power of the mind accounts for the success of any cure, whether modern surgery or carrot poultice, since few treatments work without the mind's consent and even worthless cures may work with it—witness the consistent success of the placebo effect. As Seneca observed, "The wish to be cured is part of the cure." This is the fundamental assumption of holistic health.

One problem with our attempts to stay well, be healed, or heal ourselves is that we can become obsessive about it and thus make ourselves sick. Almost all of us know at least one health fanatic who is, at worst, continuously ill with real or imagined diseases; at least, constantly involved in warding them off; and, at best, tedious company. So whatever cures you choose to take avoid the hypochondriac's pitfalls with a large dose of the following wisdom from Proverbs: "A merry heart doth good like a medicine."

CURES

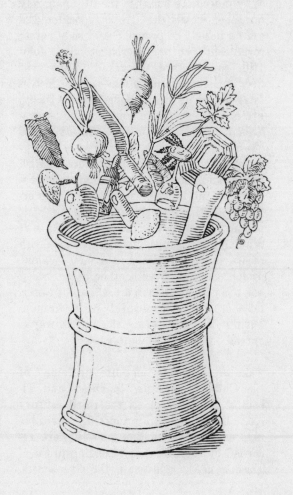

AGING

"Why should a man die if sage grows in his garden?" asks an old Arabian proverb. Why indeed. To lengthen the life span, rely on sage, which the Greeks considered a sacred herb. The proper use of sage, wrote seventeenth-century herbalist Sir John Hill, can "retard the rapid progress of decay that treads upon our heels so fast in later years of life." Sage benefits body, brain, and spirit in innumerable ways; even its official Latin name *Salvia* means "safe" or "well," indicating sage's reputation as a protector of health. As English diarist and botanist John Evelyn reported, "Tis a plant, indeed, with so many wonderful properties that the assiduous use of it is said to render men immortal." Have it regularly in soups, salads, cooked with meats and vegetables, and as a tea—alone or in combination with other herbs. Steep one teaspoon of sage in a half cup of water, let cool, and take spoonfuls of it throughout the day. Or eat sage the Italian way—spread on bread with butter.

Take ginseng, the "long-life medicine" of the Chinese, Koreans, Japanese, and Tibetans. As far back as the third century B.C. ginseng's health-promoting, revitalizing, and life-prolonging powers were recorded by the Chinese. According to them, ginseng can "rejuvenate the five senses, restore the well being of the soul, soothe fears, help cast out demons, refresh the eyes, strengthen the heart, rebuild the stamina of a bridal couple and promote the joy of productive livelihood." Its medical properties were held in such esteem that at one point in China its use was reserved for the emperor alone; he gave it to others only when their diseases would not respond to ordinary treatments. In modern-day China ginseng is still considered the medicine par excellence and is usually added to herbal prescriptions to enhance their effectiveness. It is said to rejuvenate the entire body, particularly the endocrine system, for which reason it is also known as an aphrodisiac. English poet and orientalist Sir Edwin Arnold wrote that ginseng "fills the heart with hilarity, while its occasional use will, it is said, add a decade to human life." Older people should take small doses of ginseng consistently over a long period of time. The Russians, who have done a good deal of research on it, recommend that twice a year all people over forty take ginseng daily for six consecutive weeks. Younger people should take it only occasionally and whenever they are sick or under unusual strain. It is available in teas, capsules, syrups, cordials, and the original root, which is shaped like the human body and is therefore called *ginseng*—"like a man."

Licorice is one of humanity's oldest remedies; its use as medicine dates back to

Mesopotamia where it was known as an elixir of life. The armies of the Caesars and Alexander the Great carried licorice with them on their marches as a sort of revitalizing wonder drug. And the Chinese, too, considered it a potent life sustainer and restorative, ranking its powers in this regard second only to ginseng's. You can drink water in which the desiccated roots have soaked, suck on a bit of the root or the dried cooked juice therefrom, make a tea by simmering one teaspoon of the root in a cup of boiling water, or eat real licorice candy.

Other life-lengthening substances praised by the Chinese, who were for centuries obsessed with the quest for longevity, are common yams and lettuce—though these have to be taken habitually to be effective, they note. Of these two simple vegetables, consider this: lettuce and yams were, respectively, the staple foods of 106-year-old Henry Jones and 118-year-old Dionesia Perez, consecutive holders of the title "oldest person in New York City." As for lettuce, the Roman emperor Augustus so revered its restorative, lifesaving properties that he built an altar to it and erected a statue in its honor.

According to color therapy, you can remove the ravages of time from your body and face by "breathing pink." You are supposed to visualize a lovely pink or rose-colored light surrounding you, then breathe it in deeply and slowly, sending it to your wrinkled brow or wherever its revitalizing effect is most needed. As you do this, think positive thoughts about being restored and renewed. Practice this technique for a few moments every morning and evening.

"A man can obtain longevity by sparing his ejaculation," wrote a master of the Tao of Loving. Making a distinction between orgasm and ejaculation, ancient Chinese texts say that control of ejaculation is "the single most important factor in lengthening life." Older men especially are instructed to ejaculate only rarely if they wish to retain their health, strength, and sexual vigor. The 135-year-old master Wu Tzu Tu, who learned this art at age 65, said, "All those who strive for longevity must seek it at the source of life. And the secret of this is not forcing ejaculation even when one is greatly attracted by the beauty of one's female partner. Forcing ejaculation will cause all kinds of disease." The Tao of Loving takes practice but it is said to be infinitely pleasurable, satisfying, and revitalizing to both partners.

According to European folk traditions, you may keep old age at bay by frequently inhaling the refreshing scent of rosemary —the leaves, flowers, or even the wood. As Banckes prescribed in 1525: "Make thee a box of the wood of rosemary and smell to it and it shall preserve thy youth." An old French name for rosemary is *incensier* because the herb was often burned at funerals and in sick rooms to keep away infections and assorted demons; it also repels mosquitoes.

Scandinavian legend has it that the gods eat apples to renew their youth. And the outstanding twentieth-century herbalist Maude Grieve wrote, "It is no exaggeration to say that the habitual use of apples will do much to prolong life and ameliorate its conditions." Just the smell of apples has even been said to sustain life and restore strength. So, have faith in the proverbial wisdom and eat an apple a day.

A peaceful, happy, unworried mind will do much to lengthen life, according to the tenets of Buddhist medicine. Negative emotions, say the Buddhists, such as greed, hatred, arrogance, and jealousy are very destructive and lead to physical disease and psychological strains that shorten life. It is true that most people who manage to live to a hundred or more have remarkably cheerful, relaxed dispositions.

Practice yoga postures like the shoulder stand and headstand (see page 91). They are supposed to slow down the aging process by reversing the pull of gravity on sagging flesh, putting the weight of the body instead on the pituitary, pineal, and thyroid glands, toning up these endocrine glands and thereby helping you keep the look and feel of youth. According to the more esoteric aspects of yoga, these "reverse positions" also bring about a subtle alchemical transmutation which produces an internal "elixir of life" that helps you transcend time.

Yogic breathing (see page 98) is supposed to add years to the life span since it slows down the rate of respiration—and yogis measure age in terms of breaths, not time. As one expert reported, a yogi "who could restrain his breath in this way lived . . . to an age of more than three hundred and fifty years."

If you already feel old, then heed Plato's advice and drink wine. "Wine," he wrote, "both as a sacrament and a relaxant for men of old age, was given by a god as a remedy for the austerities of old age. . . ."

If all these measures fail to delay the toll of time and the call of death, remember this from Gerard's *Herball* (1597): "For those at death's door and almost past breathing saffron bringeth breath again."

ANEMIA

Modern European and American nature healers assure us that pumpkin seeds, sunflower seeds, bran, brewer's yeast, radishes, spinach, watercress, alfalfa, almonds, raw oysters, beef liver, parsley, dried apricots and peaches, oatmeal, molasses, and cooked or liquid (but not raw) garlic will have a salutary effect on iron deficiency anemia. These foods help fight fatigue, too.

Anemic Taoists rely on date water, an easily brewed potion made by simmering whole iron-rich dates (with the pits) until a thick liquid is produced. Strain and drink a teaspoonful at a time. Date water not only helps anemia, say the Taoists, it also strengthens a weak stomach and spleen and gives you energy too. The Arabs also favor this tonic and say it cures constipation.

Take thyme freely in foods and herb teas. The Greeks believed this invigorating aromatic herb inspired courage, and the Romans used it to refresh sickly and melancholic people. Modern health experts say thyme has the effect of extracting iron from foods and making it easier for the body to assimilate. According to the late Marguerite Maury, a French biochemist and natural healer, even when taken with foods that contain no iron "thyme facilitates the formation of the red corpuscles." The Elizabethans believed a further benefit of taking lots of thyme is this: it enables you to see the fairies, who are most fond of the herb and its delightful clean scent.

According to wine therapists, persons who are anemic (though not pregnant) may treat their condition with a moderate intake of red wines, particularly French Bordeaux from Graves and Medoc, California Zinfandel, Italian Valpolicella, and Spanish sherry, since red wine has a high iron content, approximately eighty percent of which is available to the body in its soluble, or ferrous, form.

Impoverished sufferers from anemia should follow the dictates of European gypsies and American nature healers and eat copiously of young dandelion leaves—raw in salads or cooked like spinach. This wayside herb, which is free for the picking, contains valuable mineral salts believed to prevent and cure anemia, purify the blood, and normalize blood pressure.

Wealthy sufferers from anemia might try wearing rubies, as indicated by gem therapy. Rubies' hot red cosmic rays, say the gem therapists, fight tired blood.

ARTHRITIS, RHEUMATISM, ACHES AND PAINS

Consider celery. The Japanese recommend a brief mono-diet of it as a cure for all types of rheumatism, while the Chinese advocate a strong tea of celery stems for the same purpose. According to English grandmothers a glass of celery juice will perform wonders during a rheumatic attack, and gypsy women agree, adding that cucumber juice is almost as good. Modern herbalists say celery neutralizes uric acid in the body and supplies valuable minerals. Besides revering it as a panacea for arthritis, rheumatism, gout, lumbago, and neuralgia, the Chinese also believe it cures nervousness.

Keep a copper penny underfoot in your shoe or ornament yourself with a copper bracelet. Copper worn next to your skin may allay the pains of rheumatism, lumbago, sciatica, and arthritis, according to such disparate sources as American, African, Asian, and European healing systems. But why copper works is open to question. Eastern wise men say copper draws the poisons out of the body. Homeopaths explain that it keeps the body's electrical polarity in balance. When you wear copper, they say, you absorb it as a trace mineral whose function is to provide internal electrical stability and to render harmless any external electrical influences.

Furthermore, to work an optimum effect, they say it should be worn on your "negative side"—i.e., your left side if you're right-handed or vice versa. Although the copper cure was used in folk medicine for centuries, its modern use began with the discovery that African tribesmen who wore copper jewelry were remarkably free from aches and pains.

The belief of Vermont folk medicine is that bursitis, rheumatoid arthritis, osteoarthritis, and muscular rheumatism can be cured in from three to eighteen months by following this prescription: with each meal, sip a glass of water to which two teaspoons of apple cider vinegar have been added.

Wise sufferers from gouty arthritis will consume black cherries and cherry juice for quick relief. Scientific tests have indicated that cherries reduce the uric acid level in the blood. Strawberries, too, should be gobbled up. The Swedish botanist Linnaeus was the first to discover the use of strawberries as a cure for rheumatic gout. But eat them at the beginning of a meal, say the French, to draw out the body's poisons.

Folk medicine expert Lelord Kordel advises gout-ridden people to eat yogurt since its "lactic acid's" bacteria disposes of uric acid in the intestines." Kordel also reports that the Hungarian cure for gouty toe is to wrap it in a honey poultice. Because of honey's neutralizing acids, he explains, the pain is relieved within a few hours.

The Ayurvedic tradition of India prescribes watercress as the best all-purpose remedy for sciatica. Soak or cook the watercress and mix it with milk, advise the Ayurvedics. European herbalists agree that eating watercress as well as alfalfa, parsley, dandelion, and lemon can ease rheumatic pains. Homeopathic doctors caution people with rheumatism to avoid acid-forming foods such as meat, eggs, spinach, pickles, apricots, rhubarb, and tomatoes.

Modern water therapists say water can help arthritis and rheumatism. Drink large quantities of it to dissolve and remove uric acid and waste.

Afro-American and American Indian folk healers agree that the easily found, tall, tapered mullein weed provides an excellent remedy for arthritis and rheumatism and all kinds of aches, pains, sprains, and swellings, including phlebitis. Apply the fresh leaves by themselves (slip them under stockings, tee shirts, etc.) or soak a cloth in hot mullein tea and apply it to the painful area.

The nineteenth-century Irish, English, and Americans all favored potato cures for rheumatism. Carrying a potato in your pocket was a popular old-fashioned preventative measure. Reportedly even more effective was applying potato poultices—raw, peeled, and grated; or boiled and mashed, skin included—or using extremely hot potato-water baths and fomentations of hot potato water on the painful areas. The solution is made by slowly boiling down from two pints to one pint water containing one pound of quartered, unpeeled potatoes.

"Sleep with a dog to cure rheumatism," advised *The Indian Vegetable Family Instructor* in 1851. "The dog will absorb the disease and become crippled." Cruel and probably not true. A simpler, nicer way to avoid the torments of rheumatic and arthritic morning stiffness is to bed down in a sleeping bag. This has been reported to work miraculously well—the insulation from the sleeping bag retains heat and distributes it evenly throughout your body.

Bathe with roses. A handful of rose petals strewn into the tub will allay rheumatic aches and pains, say the French. In fact, they say, rose-petal baths are good for all kinds of aches and pains. For full effect, use petals that have been gathered just before the rose is about to fade.

Bathe with rosemary. And keep in mind that the ailing, failing thirteenth-century queen of Hungary, at age seventy-two, crippled with gout and rheumatism, was visited by a saintly hermit who instructed her on the mysteries of the rosemary bath. Rosemary so restored the old queen that the king of Poland fell madly in love with her and begged her to marry him.

You may soothe your pains and stimulate yourself in general by luxuriating in a warm (not hot) bath to which a sprig of rosemary or a solution of rosemary tea has been added. This bath is a reputed aphrodisiac.

Hungary water, a thirteenth-century formula named after the queen and still in use after seven centuries, is made by soaking a pound and a half of fresh rosemary tops in a gallon of spirits of wine for four days. Distill. Rub vigorously into gouty hands and feet for relief of pain.

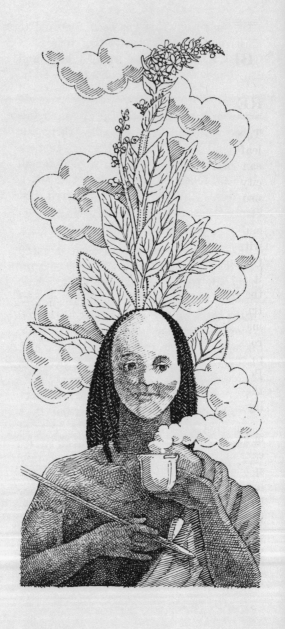

14.

ASTHMA, BRONCHITIS, COUGHS, AND RESPIRATORY AILMENTS

Take advantage of mullein, a tall, fuzzy-leafed plant that grows all over the American East and Midwest, in abandoned lots, city parks, and suburban lawns, where it is usually considered a pesty weed. The ancients, however, had a lofty respect for mullein's powers, and Odysseus carried it with him as a magical charm against Circe's enchantments. The Romans valued it for chest troubles and taught its use to the English. Numerous American Indian tribes held mullein in great esteem, primarily for the ability of its leaves and roots to relieve asthma, bronchitis, and all pulmonary complaints. The Mohican and Potawatomi tribes smoked the roots, while the Catawba boiled them and drank the liquid.

Contemporary herbalists concur that for mild respiratory problems mullein is an excellent expectorant, demulcent, and antispasmodic. The easiest way to absorb mullein's benefits, they suggest, is to steep the leaves in a teapot and inhale the fumes. Tea made from the leaves should be strained so that the leaf hairs won't tickle your throat; their fuzziness is the plant's "signature," indicating that it allays ticklish irritations of the throat and chest.

Consume garlic, honey, and onions, enduring respiratory remedies common to many far-flung healing traditions. They can be used in combination or by themselves. The use of garlic for bronchitis, asthma, and coughs due to colds dates as far back as 2000 B.C. in China. Garlic can be taken liberally without any side effects—apart from its overwhelming odor. For a cough medicine, the Chinese advise taking one teaspoon of an equal mixture of fresh garlic juice and honey throughout the day.

The Afghans use honey and garlic for asthma and bronchial infections too, while American Indian medicine men rely on garlic, honey, and onions for the same purpose. One "proven" American home remedy for asthma is to slice raw onions and top them with honey. Cover and let stand for a night. Take a teaspoon of the resultant cough syrup four times a day. Another Yankee remedy is a teaspoon of warm honey taken by itself every quarter hour. Honey is also the Romanian cure.

Consider the Siberian remedy for bronchitis: a syrup made from one part radish juice and two parts honey, a tablespoon taken before every meal and at bedtime.

The Welsh and the Hindus make a cough medicine from hot lemon juice and honey. The lemon must be baked—the Welsh fill it with honey before it goes into the oven, while the Indians mix the honey with lemon juice after heating the lemon. Roasted lemon is also said in American folk medicine to be excellent for coughs and colds.

Swallow spiderwebs, if you dare. Work up your courage by pondering the fact that the practice of swallowing a handful of spiderwebs rolled into a ball is the cure for asthma in English, European, and Australian folk medicine.

For a more orthodox aid, swallow vitamin B_6, pyridoxine. Recent scientific tests have indicated that approximately 200 mg. of it daily helps asthma sufferers, especially younger ones. Large doses of vitamin C are also said to be helpful.

Lick a licorice stick, so sweet and soothing for coughs, sore throats, mucous congestion, and all pulmonary complaints. Licorice root was mentioned for respiratory ailments as early as 2025 B.C. in Babylonia and has continued to be used for that purpose around the world up until modern times. It contains a hormone efficacious in asthma, and its natural sweetening agent (said to be fifty times sweeter than sugar) has great soothing, emollient, and demulcent properties. Richard Lucas reports that it was among the first medicinal herbs brought to America, imported by sixteenth-century English settlers who used it to overcome dry coughs, shortness of breath, and wheezing.

A licorice drink can be made by steeping or simmering the roots in water, one teaspoon rootstock per cup. That's how the ancient Egyptians drank it. If you eat licorice candy to soothe your throat, make sure it contains extract of the real stuff.

Bronchitis can provide an opportunity to indulge in a little wine therapy—in this case mulled wine. Add cinnamon, honey, cloves, and lemon peel to red wine, heat, and drink three cups a day.

Those who prefer nonalcoholic beverages might drink sunflower seed tea, a European and American folk remedy for bronchitis, pulmonary infections, coughs, and colds.

To liquify secretions in the chest, asthmatics should drink plenty of fluids, including coffee because caffeine, say modern doctors, dilates bronchial tubes and makes breathing easier. Garlic and pepper should also be taken since they help break up mucus congestion in the chest.

Japanese macrobiotic physicians say asthma can be relieved by adopting a mucusless diet: no red meat or dairy products. (This will also help cure ovarian cysts, sinus problems, prostate infections, and gallstones, they say.)

BACK TROUBLE

Use yoga to benefit your back. Almost all yoga postures have the effect of keeping the spine stretched and healthy, and yogis believe that a flexible spine keeps the aging process at bay. One of the simplest yoga techniques for the back is "rocking." It limbers up the spine and invigorates the whole system, and conquers insomnia too, they say.

Sit on a rug or mat. Draw your knees up and put your hands underneath your legs. Drop your head forward and, keeping the spine slightly rounded, use the force of your legs to propel yourself backward and forward, rocking on the ground with your spine. Do this a few times every morning.

To alleviate low-back aches, especially those caused by long hours of standing or hard work, the yoga cobra pose is recommended. It is also said to adjust displacements of the spinal column, stimulate the adrenal glands, dispel gas, and help in uterine problems and insomnia.

Lie on your stomach. Place your palms on the floor under your shoulders. Slowly inhale, look up, and raise up by rolling back your head, neck, and upper chest and using your arms to support you. The lower part of your abdomen remains on the floor and your arms partially bent. Hold your breath a few seconds while keeping your back arched. You should feel the pressure in the lower back. Then gradually begin to exhale, lowering your body slowly to the floor, uncurling your neck and head last. Rest. Repeat if you like. It's extremely easy to do.

Massaging your feet may help your back,

according to the theories of foot reflexology. Manipulate the spinal reflex in the foot (it runs along the line of the arch of the foot). Press it hard with your thumb. Rub longest on the painful points; these spots should correspond to the problem areas in your back. If this doesn't help your back, at least your feet will feel terrific.

The Center for Medical Consumers in New York City has suggested a number of things to do for your bad back, some of which are checking your posture to make sure your weight is evenly distributed, sleeping on a hard mattress in the fetal position—never on your stomach, doing some stretching exercises in the morning while still in bed, entering cars fanny first, not wearing high heels that accentuate the lumbar curve, and continuing to enjoy a normal sex life because "the exercise is good."

BAD BREATH

Mint tea "helps a stinking breath proceeding from corruption of the teeth," said Nicholas Culpeper, the seventeenth-century astrologer-physician. Rosemary, he suggested, has a similar effect. The Chinese agree on both these points. Herbalists in India recommend chewing caraway or cardamom seeds to impart a fresh fragrance to the breath.

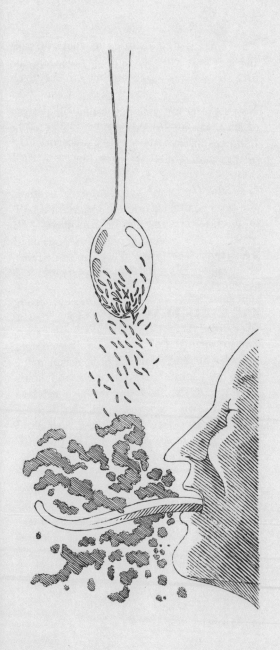

21.

To remove the offensive odor caused by eating garlic and onions, munch fresh parsley or a fresh coffee bean.

Naturopaths say you can remove one cause of halitosis by brushing the back of your tongue. (Stick out your tongue; if the root of it is coated, it needs a brushing.)

Lavender tea mouthwash and gargle (steep one teaspoon of leaves and flowers in a half to a cup of water) is a European folk remedy for sweetening the breath. It also strengthens the gums. The smell is divine and, some believe, drives away demons.

BED-WETTING

The prescription of Vermont folk medicine and the ancient Chinese is a teaspoon of honey at night. Honey attracts and holds the fluids in the body and acts as a sedative on the nervous system. And you'll probably have an easier time getting your child to take a teaspoon of honey than the anti-bed-wetting remedy that was once prevalent in Europe and among American blacks in the South: cooked mice, parboiled and fried (southern style) or roasted (continental manner). Just why mouse meat might work is something not yet comprehended.

BELCHING

Take a peel of tangerine and brew it as tea. Drink. This is the Taoist cure.

Take cucumber seeds that have been soaked and softened in water and to which a bit of saffron has been added. Eat. This is the Hindu cure.

Take a pinch of ground anise and mix it in rosewater. Drink. This is the Islamic cure.

BITES AND STINGS

Follow the advice of the Prophet Muhammad and use garlic. "In cases of stings and bites by poisonous animals, garlic acts as a theriac [sic]. Applied to the spot bitten by viper or sting of scorpion, it produces successful effects." Garlic was the preferred European medieval cure for dog bites; it is still a popular European and American remedy for wasp and bee stings.

American folk medicine prescribes putting honey on bee stings (after plucking out the stinger) or applying a handful of damp dirt or moist clay. The clay should be removed when it becomes dry and hot, then replaced with a fresh application.

BOILS AND ABSCESSES

American and Australian folk healers of the past century prescribed the same cure: covering the boil with the wet skin of a boiled egg. This, they said, is "the most efficacious remedy that can be applied to a boil," promising that it will draw off pus and relieve soreness within a few hours.

The efficacy of the fig cure is attested to in the Bible: "And Isaiah said, Take a lump of figs. And they took and laid it on the boil, and he recovered." (2 Kings 20:7) Roast and split the fig, applying the fleshy inner part to the boil. Also use it on ulcerated gums.

The homeopathic home cure is a poultice of bread or carrots. In a clean vessel, pour boiling water over slices of bread or bread crumbs and place by the fireside or near flame (not direct heat) for a few minutes. Pour off and replace with fresh boiling water two more times, then mash the bread with a fork to form the poultice. Or apply a carrot poultice made from cooked, mashed carrots.

Modern vitamin therapy suggests you fight boils with large doses of vitamin A, but as a general rule, according to the FDA and Dr. Robert C. Atkins, not more than 10,000 units a day unless under the guidance of a physician.

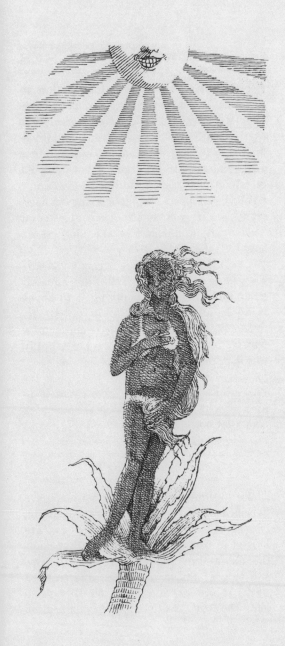

25.

BURNS

Get yourself an *Aloe vera* plant (it can be purchased at most florists) and keep it on your windowsill. The gel that oozes from the broken leaves of this succulent plant is known to be very effective in healing burns and sunburns. In addition, it can be used on all skin abrasions, irritations, wounds, wrinkles, chapped lips, bites, and even hemorrhoids. If you don't keep aloe as a houseplant, you can buy the aloe gel at health food stores.

Try using mud, as the Delaware and Algonquin Indians did, applying it to burns to "take out the fire." For immediate relief of pain, try the Victorian remedy of a tea-leaf poultice. To soothe the burn, apply raw potatoes, gobs of yogurt, or honey.

The advice given by the Red Cross is to plunge first- and second-degree burns in cold (but not icy) water.

CELLULITE

Those unsightly, dimply bulges women are horrified to find on themselves are cellulite, masses of fats, fluids, and wastes that are lodged in connective tissues and that make the outer skin (usually around the hips and thighs) pucker in a most unattractive way. According to experts on this problem, the best treatment is a purification diet high in protein and water and low in salt, plus a regimen of exercise, deep breathing, and massage. When massaging yourself, use a stroking action and always move toward the heart, pinching and kneading the problem areas for best results.

Massage therapy for cellulite may be heightened by combining it with aromatherapy. Since aromatherapy is based on the idea of treatment by osmosis, wherein, according to its French pioneer, Marguerite Maury, aromatic substances are absorbed through the skin into the ''lacunary and extracellular liquids,'' apply essential oils of juniper, lavender, or rosemary to the affected places. All of these oils are specifically prescribed for cellulite.

Aromatherapy for cellulite may be heightened by combining it with foot reflexology. Rub the essential oils into the reflex zones on the feet that ''rule'' cellulite and the lymphatic system: on the top of the feet in the spaces between the toes, especially between the big toe and second toe. Even if you haven't got any essential oils, just massage these points; according to reflexology, stimulating them helps remove the cellulite.

French healer Maurice Mességué devised a three-part treatment for cellulite. First, he advises regular massage, and second, a cleansing diet of fruits and vegetables, with plenty of natural diuretics such as onions, celery, cabbage, leeks, fennel, parsley, strawberries, and cucumbers. Cucumbers should be eaten every evening, he says, because they are a marvelous diuretic, dissolving uric acid and superfluous fat with the result that those spongy cellulite tissues "firm up wonderfully."

Third is Mességué's supreme discovery for dissolving bumpy cellulite: ground ivy, a commonly flourishing creeping (not climbing) plant that grows pretty much all over the place all year round. (And it's free.) Apply the fresh crushed ground ivy leaves to the affected parts or use a wet dressing made by dipping a towel or cloth into a solution of water in which the leaves have boiled for fifteen minutes. Also bathe your feet in this same hot solution of ground ivy "tea."

CHOLESTEROL PROBLEMS AND HARDENING OF THE ARTERIES

Wine drinking may help control cholesterol. Scientists have found that the polyphenols of red wines are a cholesterol-reducing agent. Chianti and Muscadet are said to be particularly good because of their low content of calcium salt. Unless you are pregnant, and pregnant women should drink no alcohol since it can adversely affect the fetus (and the same goes for caffeine), indulge in one to two glasses with dinner guilt free. After all, wine has been used as medicine for over four millennia. The ancient Babylonians, Egyptians, Hebrews, Hindus, Greeks, Romans, and Chinese all favored this pleasant treatment, and Louis Pasteur called wine "the most healthful, the most hygenic of beverages." Thomas Jefferson, on his doctor's order, downed a glass and a half daily.

Garlic eating, as indicated by modern laboratory tests, can help lower the level of serum cholesterol in the blood and prevent the buildup of fatty deposits on the artery walls.

Seek out sesame seeds; they have a high lecithin content, and lecithin has been shown to be especially useful in fighting hardening of the arteries. The lecithin sold in health food stores in capsules, granules, or oil is a natural derivative from soybeans, so seek out soybeans too.

CIRCULATORY PROBLEMS AND LOW BLOOD PRESSURE

For a limb that has "gone to sleep," follow these directions from the black folk medicine of the American South. Wet your second finger with spittle and make a cross on the sleeping limb to wake it up. It may be a bit esoteric, but this remedy was formerly employed in respectable British hospitals.

Add marigold flowers to your broths and salads. They are extremely cheerful and amusing when administered in this way, in addition to being excellent and a well-known folk medicine for all circulatory problems. In the Middle Ages, flowery herb salads routinely contained such healthful and delightful ingredients as marigolds, roses, violets, carnations, nasturtium, and orange blossoms.

Other simple remedies for poor circulation are: the intake of mangos, according to the Chinese; dandelions, according to the researches of Richard Lucas; thyme, which is especially good for the aged according to Carlson Wade; saffron, according to the English; ginger, according to the Japanese; and blueberries, according to French.

Jethro Kloss, perhaps America's most influential natural health healer and writer, believed poor circulation was primarily due to constipation. He therefore urged purgation of the bowels; a regimen of fresh air, exercise, and deep breathing; a cleansing diet of large quantities of fruits and vegetables; and reliance on stimulating herb teas such as red pepper (cayenne), golden seal, peppermint, spearmint, and catnip. This regimen will alleviate low blood pressure too, he said.

Ingest the B vitamin niacinamide, which is supposed to improve circulation in the extremities by dilating blood vessels there.

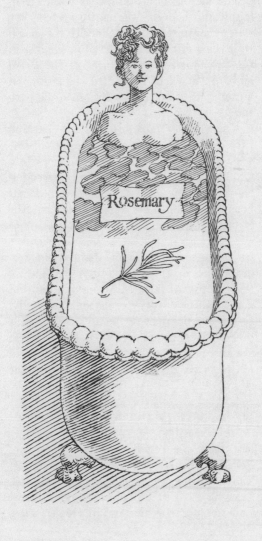

To get the old blood moving, you might try these therapeutic baths: take cold showers, cold water splashes, and cold foot baths. Cold water treatments always boost circulation and energize the entire system, say water therapists. Also bathe with rosemary, which is a stimulating herb. Put a sprig in the tub or steep two ounces of the dried leaves in a pot of hot boiled water for ten minutes, then add this solution to the bath water.

According to Japanese medicine, bathing with ginger promotes good circulation. For a ginger foot bath, grate five ounces into two quarts of hot water. Keep the feet immersed in this until they become red and hot. For a full body bath increase the amount of ginger.

Be massaged with loving hands and fragrant oils, or anoint thyself if it comes to that. Natural health enthusiasts agree that massage improves circulation markedly. Heighten its effect by using essential oils of rosemary or cinnamon, both of which are known to stimulate the circulation. Add ten to thirty drops to an ounce of massage oil.

COLDS AND FLU

For incipient colds and flu take garlic. Germs can't stand it. The Irish, Danes, Russians, Spanish, Yugoslavians, Italians, French, and Chinese all agree that liberal amounts of garlic, raw and in preparations, will prevent and cure colds and flu.

As soon as you feel the illness coming on, cook up this garlic soup, drink it, and go to bed. In half a quart of water simmer six to eight large chopped cloves of garlic with an onion or two (another traditional cold remedy known round the world) and generous portions of sage and thyme (anti-flu herbs). Season to taste with soy sauce or bouillon. You could also sip garlic tea, chew garlic cloves, or take garlic capsules, which are available in health food stores.

Use anticold and antiflu herbs. Inhaling the vapors from a simmering marjoram or oregano tea is said to afford immediate relief for aching, stuffed-up cold sufferers. Drinking teas of sage and thyme and adding these herbs to your foods will help to ward off and cure all flus and colds. Both herbs are strongly antiseptic. Thyme contains the antibacterial substance thymol, and the oils in sage have been shown to be capable of destroying bacteria, even those which resist penicillin.

You might want to follow George Washington's advice: "My own remedy," he is reported to have said, "is always to eat, just before I step into bed, a hot roasted onion, if I have a cold." The onion cure for colds, in any number of forms—soup, syrup, raw, and roasted—is centuries old and favored in Europe. Inhaling the fumes from an onion cut in half is supposed to alleviate the stuffiness of head colds.

Wear rubies or take a teaspoon of "ruby medicine water" made by steeping a ruby in a clean vessel filled with pure water. Astrologically related to the sun, rubies are supposed to release hot red cosmic rays that cure illnesses caused by cold. They are also supposed to be good for circulatory deficiencies, low blood pressure, anemia, lassitude, and stupidity. Please take off your ruby jewelry if a fever develops.

According to color therapy, you can take in the anticold red rays by eating red foods, wearing red clothes, and taking "red water medicine."

Dr. Linus Pauling recommended 2,000 mg. or more of vitamin C each day to knock out the common cold or to prevent getting it. Take 500–1,000 mg. every four hours while sick. In addition to taking vitamin C, also follow the commonsense advice from medical men and old wives: get lots of bed rest and drink lots of fluids, especially hot ones like peppermint tea, which helps raise internal heat, and hot water with lemon and honey.

In Pakistan, fresh-brewed ginger tea is taken to overcome colds and flus. Ginger is widely used around the world to counteract chills caused by dampness and frigid weather.

Eat pomegranates. The Tibetans believe they are powerful medicine and can overcome all feverish diseases caused by cold.

The fruit was a medicine of the ancient Egyptians and the ancient Greeks, who had this proverb: "Eat a pomegranate and visit a bath, your youth will haste back."

The "hot power" of red cayenne pepper is used around the world from Tibet to Africa to South America to conquer colds and flu. To avoid red pepper's biting effect on your tongue, roll some in a little bread to make an easily swallowed "pill."

To treat a common chest cold, try Granny Jeffries's English prescription that "never fails": Bake one large potato in the oven. While it cooks, liberally rub the patient's chest with goose fat (which you have cunningly saved from the Christmas roast). Remove the hot potato and put it in a woolen sock. Tie that in a rope and hang it around the sufferer's neck, so that it rests on the breast bone. Bundle up patient and potato in heavy pajamas and send off to bed.

A Jewish mother's chicken soup is great medicine once you're sick. Even modern doctors agree that the delicious salty liquid helps allay the dizziness brought on by colds and flu. Here's what you need:

   3½ to 4 pounds pullet chicken, quartered,
        including the *pupik*, liver, heart,
        and neck
     1 chicken bouillon cube (optional)
     2 to 3 quarts boiling water

1 tablespoon kosher salt
1 dash pepper
2 carrots, sliced diagonally
2 celery stalks, chopped
1 medium onion, chopped
1 bouquet of fresh parsley and dill,
  tied with a string
1 pinch nutmeg
matzoh balls made with liberal amounts
  of chicken fat

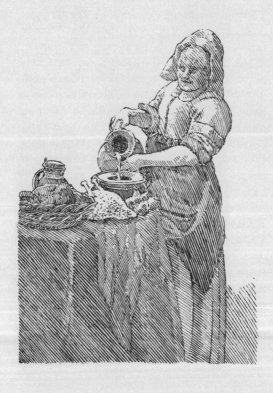

Put the chicken and bouillon into boiling water, bring to a boil again, and skim off surface scum. Add remaining ingredients except matzoh balls and partially cover. Simmer for 2½ hours. Add raw matzoh balls a half hour before soup is finished. Strain out unwanted ingredients. For best results, serve with overbearing love.

COLITIS
AND ABDOMINAL
COMPLAINTS

Why was Columbus sailing unknown seas in search of aromatic spices? Perhaps because humanity will spare no effort in its age-old attempt to settle the bowels. All the aromatic spices—nutmeg, anise, allspice, ginger, clove, cardamom, cinnamon—aid the work of the intestines and stomach.

American herbalist Benedict Lust says that in cases of colic or spasmodic pains in the abdomen, the following pleasant recipe can afford instant relief: An equal mixture of cloves, allspice, ginger, and cinnamon infused with a little brandy and warmed by the sun. A simpler but equally pleasing way to overcome abdominal pains, he says, is to drink half a pint of milk that has been boiled for ten minutes with a tablespoon of anise seeds.

Garlic, which the Roman naturalist Pliny prescribed for sixty-one disorders of the body, can be an aid in intestinal disorders.

Nearly two thousand years later it is still said to promote the functioning of the intestines, fight colitis and dyspepsia, and relieve gas and constipation. Scientific research has shown that daily garlic intake actually changes the composition of the intestinal flora, benefiting the "good bacteria" and decreasing the harmful bacteria there.

Yogurt also promotes the growth of helpful intestinal flora, and has been used as an intestinal preventative and combative folk medicine since biblical times. It should especially be consumed whenever you have had to take antibiotics like penicillin or tetracycline, since antibiotics destroy all bacteria, including the "good" kinds.

According to wine therapy, warm ruby red wines—particularly Bordeaux—should be taken by colitis sufferers to allay the intestinal cramps of colic and increase the calcium in the bloodstream. But you must drink them warmed (not room temperature) if you want to get the full medicinal effect.

Grape diets can be an amazing help. Herbalist Ben Charles Harris explains that grapes "are alkaline and mineral rich fruits" that "help the body rid itself of accumulated poisons." Grapes are said to rejuvenate the entire digestive tract and detoxify the body. For one thing, as folk medicine expert Lelord Kordel explains,

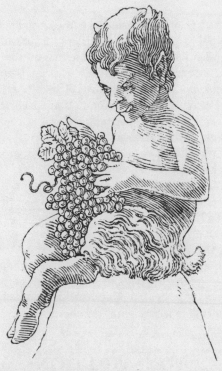

grapes, which ferment rapidly, "impart their fermentation to other foods, releasing alcohol and poisons into the bloodstream." For another, as recent Canadian research has shown, grapes are positively lethal to viruses. A one to three day "grape fast" (two to four pounds of grapes per day with some milk, yogurt, and whole grain allowed if you like) is said to have great health benefits and has been used by people all over the world as a curative measure. Some people have even claimed that grape fasts can cure cancer.

In addition, you can get the benefit of grapes from grape poultices, as recommended by American psychic diagnostician and natural healer Edgar Cayce. Grape packs, said Cayce, can cure colitis, gastritis, intestinal gas, and elimination problems as well as pelvic and glandular disorders, rheumatism, tumors, incoordination, and ulcers. You may use the grape pack alone without going on a grape fast.

Mash grapes—skin, seed, and all—of any type, although the Concord variety is preferred, and wrap the grape mush in a layer of muslin, linen, or bed sheet. Lay it on the affected part for an hour or two, and apply a fresh pack after the first hour. Use for three days and wait a week before beginning again. Cayce recorded phenomenal success with this unusual treatment.

CONSTIPATION

Liberated from Victorian constraints in the bedroom? Then liberate yourself from Victorian practices in the bathroom, namely the toilet seat. The Victorians preferred the toilet seat as an esthetic improvement over the natural squatting position used by the "primitive world," but the squat puts pressure on the abdominal muscles and the intestines and acts as a natural stimulant to defecation. You can squat on a toilet; it just takes a little practice.

Try this morning routine: first thing, drink some water, preferably boiled (see page 72). You may add a little honey to it if you like. Water taken on an empty stomach stimulates peristalsis by reflex, says Dr. Jacques Thiroloix, a constipation expert. And honey is said to be a natural laxative.

Down one tablespoon of olive oil every morning before breakfast, as people do in Mediterranean countries. Olive oil is an ancient cure for constipation, and consuming it in the morning not only helps the bowels to move but also gets the liver and gallbladder working. The lighter-colored, usually more expensive olive oils taste much better than the darker, cheaper kinds. Add a few drops of fresh lemon to it if you find the taste too bitter.

What modern processing took away, modern medicine now says to put back: bran, the fibrous coating lost in the processing of white flour. Our fiber-free, fast-food diet has ruined our intestines, but all we have to do is take two to three tablespoons of bran every morning and the bran fiber will help normalize bowel function. It should be the raw, unprocessed bran, not the commercial cereal variations. Sprinkle on other cereal. In general, always use whole grains instead of refined ones.

41.

Nibble on prunes (traditional American cure), rhubarb jam (French cure), ripe papayas (Chinese cure), and lots of raw green vegetables, fresh fruits, and soured milk products like yogurt and buttermilk (modern nutritionists' cure).

CORNS

Thrust your toe into a lemon and in this manner go to bed for the night. According to Euro-American folk medicine, two or three nights spent with a lemon on the toe will easily remove even the worst corns. In Sri Lanka, they slice the lemon and place it over the corn.

At age 106, Henry Jones could still find medicine growing everywhere he went, even in New York City, an art he learned from his aunt, a maid on President Carter's peanut plantation. Asked for a remedy for corns, he replied, "Take mullein, the gray grass that grows free for the pickin' in Central Park. Heat it in hot water, put your feet in it up to your ankles. It pulls the dead load. Don't burn you. No trouble to you."

DANDRUFF

The medieval health handbook *Tacuinum Sanitatis*, which experts believe to be a thirteenth-century Latin translation of a work by a tenth-century Arabian physician, says simply that beet juice eliminates

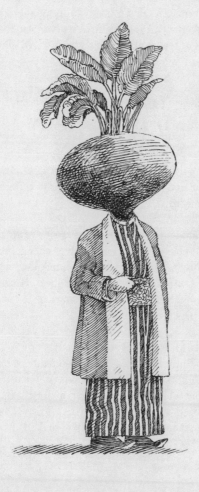

dandruff. To this day the Arab remedy for dandruff remains washing the hair with beet juice mixed with water and a little salt. Can a thousand years of use of something that is terribly messy and stains not work? This is best for brunettes since beet is a dye.

In India and Pakistan, the juice of fresh marijuana leaves is used to remove dandruff. American nature healers suggest that cool sage tea makes a most effective hair tonic and gets rid of dandruff.

DIARRHEA
AND DYSENTERY

The number one cure from Asia is unrinsed boiled white rice, a sticky, gummy mass of carbohydrates that may quickly plug you up.

Take jams and compotes of roses, quince, and blueberries. Laboratory experiments have shown that blueberry juice destroys some harmful intestinal microbes. Herbal traditions agree that the berries furnish one of the best specifics against diarrhea.

Many Indian Ayurvedic remedies for diarrhea include bananas, which contain pectin and promote the growth of beneficial intestinal bacteria. Three times a day eat a well-boiled unripe banana that has soaked in yogurt or a ripe banana soaked in a cup of milk. For dysentery Ayurvedic healers prescribe hot lemon water.

When eating strawberries, save the leaves. According to naturopaths, a tea made from steeping them in boiled water helps diarrhea and various types of bowel troubles. Peppermint tea is also said to help, and so is carrot soup.

DRUNKENNESS AND ALCOHOLISM

Desperation with drunken friends and family may drive you to follow this occult remedy from the Pennsylvania Dutch: "If you scrape the dirt collected under [the drunkard's] fingernails and put some into whiskey which the drunkard will gladly drink, it will cure him of his nasty habit."

To "delay drunkenness" consume sweet almonds before imbibing, as did merrymakers in the Middle Ages. The belief that eating almonds on an empty stomach prevents intoxication later can be traced back to the ancients and is the probable origin of the modern custom of munching salted almonds with cocktails. Taken before a belt of booze, almonds are said to have the additional advantage of preventing anxiety.

The miracle of honey yet again. "Honey counteracts the craving for alcohol and successfully accomplishes the sobering-up process," says Dr. Jarvis from his experiences with drunken Vermont folks. He suggests giving repeated teaspoonsful of honey in the first stages of the sobering-up process —one every few minutes, increasing the dosage to six teaspoonsful every twenty minutes. In this manner, with the help of two pounds of honey, a paralyzed drunk may be transformed into an upstanding citizen in twenty-four hours.

If the alcoholic habit is truly tormenting, try the appropriately tormented nineteenth-century French cure for perpetual drunkenness: drink the blood of a mole.

EAR AILMENTS

For deafness and noise in the head, a widely used cure in nineteenth-century England and America was to place a few drops of urine in the ears.

According to Indian Ayurvedic medicine, you may cure earaches by inserting a peeled clove of garlic into the ear. The American home cure is similar, but adds that the garlic should be steeped in warm olive oil for a few minutes, then rolled into a small piece of fine linen before placing in the ear. Plug ear with cotton after removing.

A roasted onion applied warm to the ear is a remedy for earache common to America, Europe, and Africa.

EYE AILMENTS

Parsley has the power to cure eye inflammations and conjunctivitis, according to French and English herbalists. The leaves can be laid on inflamed or swollen eyes, or a fomentation of cooled parsley tea can be applied with cotton.

Longfellow wrote:

> Above the lower plants it towers,
> The Fennel with its yellow flowers;
> And in an earlier age than ours
> Was gifted with wondrous powers
>   lost vision to restore.

Pliny, the second-century Roman naturalist, recommended fennel as a cure for failing eyesight, and belief in this remedy has persisted through the centuries. In our own times it is still widely recommended by herbalists as an excellent wash for sore, irritated, and strained eyes; and Jethro Kloss says that taken internally it will benefit the eyes and strengthen them.

For a tea, steep one teaspoon of crushed fennel seeds in water for five minutes, strain, and drink. Dilute this one third with water for an eyewash.

The Tibetans believe moon gazing strengthens the vision and cools overheated, inflamed eyes. Gaze moonward for ten to twenty minutes, especially when the moon is full. They also prescribe fennel.

William Bates, a bold American ophthalmologist of this century, stated that contrary to popular medical opinion weak vision can be improved with eye exercises. Dr. Bates observed that, after all, the eye is a muscle and is subject to muscle strain. His system of visual reeducation is based on relaxation, and one of its simplest techniques is called palming. Cover your closed eyes completely with your hollowed palms (no pressure on the eyes), fingers crossed over the forehead. You can rest your elbows on something in front of you so that your back and neck stay straight. Remain in the soothing darkness for a few minutes using your "inner vision" to imagine peaceful vistas and pleasant surroundings.

When you uncover your eyes, the habit of straining temporarily forgotten, you may see the world very clearly for a moment.

To relieve itching or to remove foreign substances from one eye, try this magic remedy from the Pennsylvania Germans: rub the other eye. This cure is supposed to work by "sympathetic reaction."

Marijuana proponents claim their favorite weed, smoked or eaten, relieves the intraocular pressure of glaucoma. Some scientific research backs up this theory. The trouble with the cure is that it's illegal.

According to traditional American folk medicine, applications of cool, damp tea bags reduce the swelling of puffy eyes,

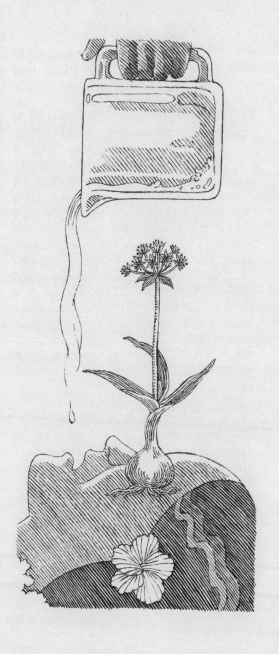

49.

slices of cucumber soothe strained eyes, and cooled camomile tea eyewashes alleviate conjunctivitis.

According to Maurice Mességué, eating blueberries helps improve night blindness.

The psychic readings of Edgar Cayce revealed the usefulness of the following exercises for all vision problems. Sit or stand with your back straight, then bend your head forward three times, back three times, to the right three times, and to the left three times. Follow this by slowly rolling your head clockwise three times and counterclockwise three times. These exercises must be done morning and evening to achieve better vision, said Cayce. Furthermore, he advised cataract sufferers to do them patiently for six months, after which time he predicted the cataracts would improve markedly.

The dry yellow husks of *aka'aku'* (otherwise known as onions) are great for the eyes, according to the practical folk medicine of Hawaii. Boil a handful of the clean husks in water, cool, strain, and drink "a little bit every day to give strength to the eyes."

FEMALE COMPLAINTS

To regulate the menstrual flow and relieve suppressed menses, the Persian and French remedy is a few cups of fennel tea (steep the bruised seeds in boiled water); the American folk cure is ginger tea. Modern herbalists say that women troubled with irregular menstruation will benefit from taking a tea of marjoram three or four days before the period is due.

To bring on suppressed menses, according to European herbalism, drink teas of sweet basil, sage, rosemary, or thyme. The last was known in olden days as mother thyme because of its salutary influence on the womb.

For menstrual cramps and premenstrual nervousness drink catnip tea. Culpeper

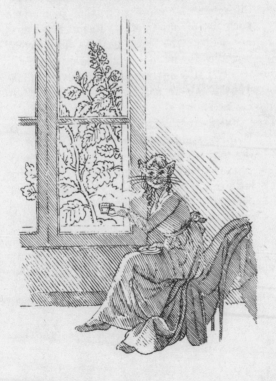

calls it an herb of Venus, and adds that its frequent use "taketh away barrenness." Pour a pint of boiling water over two teaspoons of catnip. Steep for five minutes.

Herbs said in many quarters to help foster conception are motherwort, lavender, chicory, raspberry leaf, red clover, lettuce, feverfew, sage, watercress, and catnip— which the Afgans primarily rely on. Take these alone or in combinations as tea.

A panacea during pregnancy is raspberry leaf tea. It is supposed to do everything from allaying morning sickness to preventing miscarriage to easing labor pains. One herbalist of old wrote: "Raspberry leaves are one of the most useful and efficient remedies for women in labour, quieting untimely pains but rendering them more efficient if labour has really commenced." It has no known side effects.

Raspberry leaf tea was widely used by English women in the Midlands and West Country and in this century even officially employed in the Worcestershire maternity hospitals. Pour one pint of boiling water over two teaspoonsful of the leaves and steep for five minutes.

During pregnancy and lactation Mexican women drink large quantities of orange juice. They believe it rids the body of harmful poisons.

The sore, swelled, or caked breasts of the

nursing mother can be relieved, according to an American midwife of the last century, by applying hot pancakes made of sour milk, baking soda, and wheat flour. The pancakes should be large enough to cover the entire breast and should be replaced before becoming cold. For cracked nipples, apply molasses. To keep the milk flowing, eat carrots. To help stop the flow of milk, the nineteenth-century herb expert Fernie recommended sage tea.

Garden peas may prove contraceptive. English physician William Thompson reports that garden peas caused a loss of fertility in laboratory rats. You might also try eating yams. The steroids of modern birth control pills come primarily from them. Mexican women believe yams have an overall beneficial and regulating effect on the female reproductive system.

If you have made love without using birth control but really don't want to conceive, you could try this Arab trick, although only on the theory that at some point anything is better than nothing: bound out of bed and jump up and down with all your might eight or nine times "to cause the seminal fluid to fall down from the mouth of the womb."

To combat the "yeast" type of vaginal infection, some people recommend that yogurt containing the live acidophilus culture be applied to the irritated parts and used as a douche. Yeast infections can also be treated in early stages, according to modern gynecologists, by using a douche of two to three teaspoons of baking soda in two quarts of water.

For trichomonas infections, before they become acute, douche with two to three tablespoons of white vinegar in two quarts of warm water. In general, avoid nylon underpants and panty hose, because they retain heat and moisture, which aggravate vaginal infections.

A variety of menopausal problems may be helped by sage tea. Sage is said to be a tonic to the uterus and to have a regulating effect on the hormones, which makes it good to use during puberty and pregnancy also.

For excessive menstrual flow during the change of life, the American folk prescription is to take, three times a day, one teaspoon of a cordial made from an ounce of fresh ground nutmeg mixed in a pint of Jamaican rum.

For the headaches and hot flashes of menopause, Sarah Beckett, a specialist in herbs for feminine ailments, recommends saffron tea. Steep one teaspoon in a pint of water, cool, strain, and take three teaspoonsful per day.

FEVER

A colonial fever remedy adapted from American Indian medicine is magnolia bark, particularly the root bark, boiled in wine or infused in brandy. This extraordinary beverage was also used for all types of internal pains and dysentery.

Feverish teetotalers should opt for onions, a favorite cure in Europe and early America. Slice onions and bind them to the soles of the feet to draw out the fever. For children, use sliced potatoes instead.

Somewhat crude and difficult to procure, but who knows, perhaps all the more effective for the trouble, is the Kansas, Texas, and Minnesota folk remedy for reducing temperatures: jackrabbit turd tea. The Texans maintain that the bunnies' droppings must be kept throughout one winter in an airtight jar, after which time they may be brewed into a strong medicinal tea—please strain it before drinking. Minnesotans say the tea can be made directly after the droppings are collected. In any case, they all believe this strange brew "never fails" to break the fever.

Is turd medicine odd, disgusting, and absolutely out of the question? Martin Luther didn't think so: "Swine's dung stints the blood; horse's serves for pleurisy," he said, adding that "man's heals wounds and black blotches."

If you can't stand the sight or scent of dung, you may prefer the pleasant remedy of the Australian Aborigines who use eucalyptus leaves to fight fevers. Their wisdom in this matter proved so effective that their remedy was widely absorbed into the folk medicine of Australian whites. Eucalyptus oil is known for its pronounced cooling effect and its ability to reduce temperature. You can get eucalyptus leaves from a florist (or from trees in the forests of California). Crush a few leaves and inhale their camphoraceous odor, rub the crushed leaves on the temples and forehead, or drop the crushed leaves in boiling water and inhale the steam.

While lying around prostrate with fever, sip lots of fluids, especially Earl Grey tea. It's flavored with bergamot oil, the Italian folk remedy for reducing temperatures.

West Indian medicine men cure red-hot fevers with hot red peppers. Although it might seem contradictory, red pepper's effect is cooling. The West Indians drink it as a tea, mix it with orange juice, or chew the pods raw (which you may not quite be up to). In fact, the West Indians use it as a panacea against most maladies and as a main preventative medicine.

Use your tongue to cool your body. All you have to do is practice *sitali kumbhaka,* a yogic imitation of the respiration of the serpent. Stick out the tongue and curl the sides to make a "tube." Draw in the air through the mouth making the hissing sound *se.* Hold as long as possible and exhale through the nose. Do fifteen to thirty times a day. It will cool you off.

FLATULENCE

Fight gas with anise seeds, as the American Indians did. One tribe named the seed *Tut-Te-See-Hau*, "it expels the wind." You can chew the other carminative seeds like caraway or fennel (which most Indian restaurants thoughtfully provide after a meal) for the same effect. Also, drink teas of carminative herbs such as ginger, coriander, camomile, and peppermint.

Infants who are suffering from gas can be given the age-old English folk cure of dill tea. "The name dill," wrote British herbalist Eleanour Rohde, "is supposed to be derived from the Saxon *dillian*—to lull, because a decoction was made from the seeds to soothe babies to sleep." Dill water is still listed today in *British Pharmacological Index* for "treatment of flatulence in infants."

Try the "wind-removing" pose of yoga. Lie flat on your back. Inhale deeply, expanding the abdomen. Hold the breath and draw up your knees toward your chest, hold them there with your hands, and press your abdomen against the folded legs. Exhale and release legs. Repeat until you get the desired relief.

Also try the "rabbit" pose. Stand erect, inhale into abdomen, extend arms straight out in front of you and bend at the knees, keeping the back straight. Tighten abdomen muscles. You now look like a rabbit about to pass gas. Do these exercises in private.

FROSTBITE

Do as the Red Cross advises: have a warm drink, bundle up, do not rub the affected part, but put it in warm (not hot) water.

Nineteenth-century American wisdom advised binding the frostbitten parts with a poultice of roasted turnips.

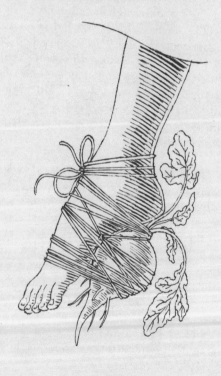

GALLSTONES

Don't leave that parsley garnish on your plate. Eat it up and all the other parsley you can get—raw, in soups, juices, and tea. What we clever moderns perceive as a lowly green hardly fit to be eaten the ancient Greeks considered sacred. In centuries past it acquired the nickname parsley break-stone because of its peculiar power to dissolve gallstones as well as urinary and kidney gravel. So drink infusions of it as often as you can, preferably following the advice of natural medicine expert Dr. H. E. Kirschner who says that adding boiled onions to a parsley brew makes it an even more effective gallstones fighter.

Drink camomile tea, which Culpeper claimed could dissolve gallstones.

GRAYING HAIR

According to shiatsu massage from Japan, you may prevent your hair from turning gray by regular finger pressure on the three points in the front of your neck on each side of your thyroid gland, which is beneath the Adam's apple. With the thumb of your right hand press each point on the right side for two seconds, then release. Repeat five times, then switch to the left side and repeat the whole procedure. Shiatsu master Tokujiro Namikoshi says this will have the added effect of beautifying your skin because it stimulates the production of hormones.

If you are mystically inclined but still vain enough to care whether you turn gray, then heed this advice from Islamic holy men as recorded by Arabic medicine expert Robert Thompson: Have date jam for breakfast every morning for a month, and during the last week of that period drink water gathered from a holy shrine (they prefer sacred Moslem places, but you may choose whatever water you have faith in). For the next month go without sex and sour food, then take a purgative to cleanse your system. In this way your heart will be pure, your soul will be white, and your hair may be dark again.

The Chinese believe that applying a combination of ground cloves and fresh ginger juice to the scalp will prevent the hair from turning gray.

HAIR LOSS

According to reflex therapy, you may prevent yourself from going bald by rubbing the fingernails of one hand across those of the other with a buffing motion, for five minutes a day.

Onions on the scalp have a long history of fighting baldness. From the Middle Ages

to the present day they have been prescribed to stimulate hair growth. Try
rubbing the bald part with an onion in the
morning and evening till the scalp turns
red, then rubbing it with honey. Or try
preventing baldness with a daily scalp
massage of diluted onion juice mixed with
a little honey. Some say these measures will
also darken gray hair.

Baldness may be kept at bay by standing
on your head (see page 91), which will
provide oxygen to the "oxygen-choked"
hair bulbs. Health expert Carlson Wade
explains that "sufficient oxygen is vital to
help rejuvenate the scalp and promote hair
growth."

Supplements of the B vitamins and vitamin
E may help prevent and control baldness,
according to modern nutritional therapists.

HANGOVER

To settle the upset stomach of early morning hangover (otherwise known as alcoholic gastritis), the Chinese prescribed a
cup of ginger tea.

Follow this advice from a nineteenth-
century medicine manual: "To remove the
effects produced by an excess of wine, etc.,
drink a wineglassful of olive oil. It will
prevent the hurtful fumes from rising. It
will have the same effect if taken before
an intended debauch."

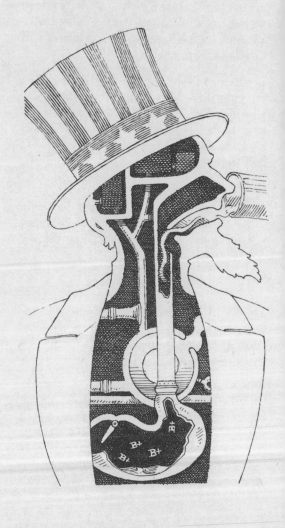

Follow this hangover advice from wild-herb stalker Euell Gibbons: Drink thyme tea with lots of honey and a touch of salt. Or, try the West Indian hangover remedy: cayenne pepper, straight or as tea.

The modern American cure is to take several B complex vitamins and a large glass of water before going to bed or, if you are too far gone for that, when you get up.

According to hand reflexology, you can relieve the pounding of a hangover headache by massaging your thumbs with the index finger and thumb of the opposite hands. Furthermore, according to Chinese acupressure, you can relieve pain in the eyes, ears, nose, teeth, mouth, and brain (all of which are known to carry on terribly during hangovers) by pinching and kneading the important *ho-ku* acupuncture point in the inner upper part of the web between the forefinger and thumb. You can locate it by bringing your thumb close into the edge of your hand; it's the high fleshy part of the ridge formed there. Massage it with the thumb and forefinger of the opposite hand.

HAY FEVER

The American frontier hay fever cure is the inhalation of coffee fumes. Heat fresh coffee grounds on hot coals and heartily whiff in the resulting smoke.

Vermont folks put their faith in the honey-bee, using honeycomb as a desensitizing, antiallergic agent for hay fever. As a preventative measure, chew honeycomb once a day for a month before the hay fever season arrives. If it is already upon you, then chew honeycomb three times a week or take two teaspoons of honey with each meal. Increase the dosage for more severe cases. The U.S. Army tested this cure and found many individuals got great relief from it, especially from chewing the honey-combs.

HEADACHE

Place an ironed cabbage leaf on your forehead. If you think you'd feel ridiculous doing this, think how people like Pope John XXIII, Winston Churchill, Jean Cocteau, or King Farouk must have felt when they went to French nature healer Maurice Mességué for a cure and got cabbage. Cabbage, says Mességué, is an "ideal first aid material" and a universal panacea for so many ailments. It has the unique ability to draw out pain. For headaches, including migraines, his prescription is to take a large, fresh leaf and cut out the central rib. Iron the leaf to make it soft or achieve the same effect by dipping the leaf in boiling hot water or letting it soak in olive oil overnight. Place it on the brow or wherever the pain is located. Relax and experience the miracle of cabbage.

Bind fresh mint to your forehead and lie down. Or place a warm mint compress on your brow, made by dipping a towel into a very strong infusion of mint tea. Drink some peppermint tea as well. Mint is a foremost headache cure in the herbal medicine traditions of Europe and America.

Snuff out your headache in the English way. Sir John Floyer, seventeenth-century physician to Charles II, wrote this of his favorite headache remedy: "the juice of Ground-ivy snuft up into ye nose out of a spoon taketh away ye greatest paine thereof that is. This medicine is worth gold." Ground ivy grows freely over most of America.

For headaches from nerves, hangovers, and poor circulation, rosemary tea has been recommended for centuries. And most twentieth-century herbalists, including Maude Grieve, Jethro Kloss, Joseph Kadams, Ben Charles Harris, and the two Lusts (uncle Benedict and nephew John) agree it works.

Contemporary Chinese acupressure therapy for headaches consists of first massaging the temples and the point between the brows to loosen them up, then using the "wiping massage technique" (pulling your finger hard) from the point between the brows straight up the forehead to one inch above the hairline; follow with the wiping technique from the point between the brows out to the temples. Do these alternating strokes twenty to thirty times each.

HEART DISEASE AND BLOOD CLOTS

Jog. Run in place. Do it however you like, but make sure you do some exercise every day to give a good workout to your heart and lungs. New studies have suggested that running and jogging really do curb heart disease. Runners had a higher blood level of HDL, a substance associated with reduced rate of coronary disease, than nonexercisers. If you've been a nonrunner and nonmover for a long time, build up your heart strength gradually by beginning a gradual exercise program; otherwise, if you suddenly get up and run around the block after not having moved for years, it may be too much for your body and your heart.

Dine on onions if you have coronary problems or a tendency toward blood clots. Eating fried or boiled onions provides protection against blood clots and helps to dissolve them, according to the French and the Chinese. And because of the success some French people had in using onions to treat blood clots in horses, researchers were spurred on to test onions scientifically. They discovered that onions increase fibrinolytic activity in the blood. Russian scientists have shown that onions are good for all kinds of heart trouble—weak hearts, high blood pressure, hardening of the arteries, and poor circulation.

A bit of champagne may be sipped gaily with the knowledge that because of its rich tartrate of potassium content, it has a positive effect on muscle strength and contractility and hence on cardiac rhythm, or so say the wine therapists. A moderate intake of alcohol, it has been reported by researchers, also helps increase the body's level of HDL, and so helps prevent heart disease. So do have some.

If you can't get champagne, try dry, light white wines, which are especially recommended for people with hypertension. Please remember, however, that alcohol is never recommended for women who are pregnant.

Eat wheat germ for a healthy heart. According to health writer Linda Clark, "there is laboratory proof that this simple, natural food substance can be a remedy for heart disease. . . ." Wheat germ, like bran, has been removed from the modern diet by "sophisticated" food processing and refining, but it contains large amounts of vitamin E, which has been used successfully to treat heart disease. One Canadian doctor has stated that prior to the removal of wheat germ from our food at the beginning of the century "there were no cases of coronary thrombosis."

Sip peppermint tea often, as Russian peasants have been doing for centuries. Russian folk medicine prescribes it as an excellent tonic for all heart afflictions, including palpitations. Sweeten it with honey, which some British physicians say is great for weak hearts and general physical repair.

The English call dandelion "heart fever grass" because of its beneficial action in heart disease. Try eating raw dandelion leaf salad or drinking dandelion tea.

Because their color symbolizes blood, red roses have been prescribed to strengthen the heart, purify the blood, overcome dizziness, and help in disorders of the liver, gallbladder, and stomach. Consume their red petals raw, in jams, as tea, or in a compote cooked with honey and apple juice (remove the bottom white part of the petal —it's bitter).

In Asia and Europe the rose has been appreciated not only for its beauty and romance and the power of its sweet scent but also as a supreme medicine. Roses are said to make the heart merry and keep the vital spirits lively. In India some tribes of wandering mystics live on roses alone, while the Persian philosopher Zarathustra spoke thusly of them: roses are the mother of all nutritious food. For one thing, they contain large amounts of vitamin C.

HEMORRHOIDS

The following exercise will clear up hemorrhoids, according to psychic diagnostician Edgar Cayce. Raise the hands high above the head, then bend forward to bring the hands as close to the floor as possible. Repeat for two or three minutes morning and evening. Furthermore, patients who followed Cayce's famous almond-eating dic-

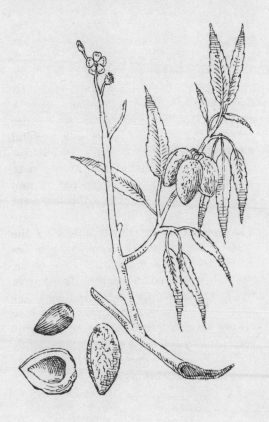

tum ("three almonds a day keep cancer away") reported that it also cleared up their piles.

Known as "the sleeping prophet" because he received his healing knowledge while in a state of deep trance, Cayce had remarkable success with his treatments.

For bleeding piles, you might try this recipe from India and Pakistan. Apply a paste of powdered sesame seeds that have been mixed with water and a little sweet oil.

HICCUPS

Put your hiccups in the bag, literally. Place a brown paper bag (no plastic, please) over your head, just like a child's mask. Inhale and exhale for a few minutes. The resultant accumulation of carbon dioxide may stop the spasms (so may the absurdity of sitting around in this manner).

The American folk remedy is to let a teaspoon of sugar dissolve on your tongue. The English folk cure is to drink a tea of dill seeds. Hindu medicine suggests that you alternately drink cups of hot and cold milk until the hiccups disappear. Drinking orange juice has been said to be an almost certain cure. One American nineteenth-century doctor suggested sticking your tongue out and keeping it there.

HIGH BLOOD PRESSURE AND HYPERTENSION

What the yogis have claimed to work for centuries has now been proved by medical science, so you might as well learn how to do it: relax and meditate. The British medical journal *Lancet* recently announced that yoga and meditation may soon become the regular form of treatment for hypertension, and some physicians have claimed that yogic breathing can normalize hypertension within three weeks. So try either of the simple forms of meditation described here or yogic breathing, which is described on page 98).

The first meditation technique is counting your breath. Breathe normally, as opposed to yogic deep breathing, concentrating pointedly on the process of breathing and on counting the exhalations. Silently count up to five, then start over again, and continue in this way. If you lose track, begin again with one. Just maintain your awareness, keep breathing, and keep counting.

The second meditation technique is concentration on the repetition of a mantric sound. You repeat the ancient mantra OM AH HUM, chanting it slowly, gently, and softly, or even inaudibly to yourself, if you prefer, focusing all your attention on it. Center your awareness on this mantra and completely relax in and with it.

Always do meditation in a relaxed sitting position, keeping the back straight. Decide on a time period—five to ten minutes at first, then twenty minutes to a half hour —even set a timer if you have one. Besides lowering your blood pressure, meditation can be enlightening.

In distant and present time garlic has been recommended as a cure for high blood pressure. Legend has it that an ancient emperor of China cured himself of hypertension by the use of garlic. Modern natural health proponent Gary Null says garlic use brings clearly measurable improvements in high blood pressure and has a dilating effect on the blood vessels. Evidence to this effect comes from scientific research in Switzerland, Germany, and India. Onion eating has a similar effect, according to the Russians.

INDIGESTION AND STOMACH AILMENTS

For chronic indigestion, and the host of disorders stemming from it, try the simplest remedy of all—boiled water. According to the Buddhists, boiled water was the first medicine, prescribed by the Medicine Buddha himself. But if you don't believe the Buddhists, ponder the fact that this remedy has been known and practiced around the world since the dawn of time. Remember that the Father of Western medicine, Hippocrates, used boiled water to treat innumerable disorders. And then consider the case, in 1897, of an American man whose digestive system was so faulty that he was given up to die. He heard of the boiled water cure from a German doctor, took it up, and was saved from death and a sour stomach. So learn the procedure, which is as follows:

In the morning before taking any other food or beverage, boil water for a minimum of five minutes but preferably for twenty, at which point all the parasites are killed, and the water is "alchemically transformed" into its pure nature—that length of boiling certainly gives it a clean, sweet taste. Then drink it. You can cool it slightly and replace the oxygen lost in the boiling process by pouring it back and forth a few times between two cups. Hot boiled water is a remarkably satisfying beverage.

Among its many benevolent qualities, sage is strongly antiseptic; it is also stimulating in debility of the stomach and weakness of the digestion generally. For these and other reasons the Chinese prized it highly. In fact they thought the early Dutch traders fools to trade sage for three times its amount in Chinese black tea, since through repeated use, sage tea helps while the black tea hurts.

The French take sage in wine and also use sage in food to avoid digestive problems. Added to meat dishes during their cooking, sage is said to prevent putrefaction. Thyme is also used by the French as an excellent remedy for difficult digestion and tired intestines. Use it freely.

Basil is a stomach settler. It may, like sage, be added to white wine and taken after meals. When added to food during the cooking process, it makes it more digestible. When added to salads, says French biochemist–natural healer Marguerite Maury, its antiseptic qualities remove the multitude of contaminations fresh foods are heir to. Basil has an antispasmodic effect on the stomach, aids digestion in general, and even helps against constipation. This sacred herb of the Hindus is believed to protect all who grow it or keep it nearby.

Those afflicted with indigestion should drink white wines, which act as a natural stimulant on the gastric juices and are therefore helpful to dyspeptic people. Take note, however: to combat indigestion white wines should be drunk at the end of meals, not with them.

"No simple remedy in the whole catalogue of herbal medicine is possessed of a quality more friendly and more beneficial to the intestines than chamomile flowers," wrote Dr. Fernie in 1897. Camomile tea is used throughout southern Europe as a remedy for stomachaches, abdominal pains, flatulence, and poor digestion, especially for children, convalescents, and the aged.

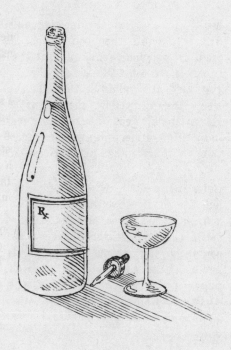

When a bit of ginger is added to it, it proves even more settling. Mint tea is also wonderful in this regard, as is cinnamon.

Hawaiians, Polynesians, and other Asian peoples depend on papaya for dyspepsia. Papaya contains an enzyme called papain, similar to pepsin, which performs miracles for the digestion, breaking down foods to a digestible state. Even the U.S. Department of Agriculture lauds papaya's "peculiar and valuable digestive properties." Expensive pills called papaya enzyme are sold in health food stores as digestive aids, but why take a pill when you can eat this incredibly delicious fruit and get the same beneficial results? Make sure the papayas you buy are yellow rather than green; when they're yellow they're ripe. The Hawaiians also eat pineapples to overcome indigestion. Pineapples, like papayas, contain an enzyme that helps digest protein.

Color therapists insist that yellow is excellent for all digestive disorders of the stomach, intestines, liver, and gallbladder. You can absorb yellow's healing rays, they are convinced, by eating yellow foods like lemons, bananas, grapefruit, squash, and papayas; by wearing yellow clothes; by massages with "yellow potenized oils," and by drinking "yellow potenized" water.

When afflicted with heartburn, whatever you do, don't lie down. Remember this sensible advice from modern medicine: remain upright, thus preventing the backflow of acid from the stomach.

All fat, lethargic, and sickly types who are plagued with chronic disorders of the digestive system should follow the example of Horace Fletcher. In 1898, at age forty, Horace was overweight and subject to constant colds, fatigue, and indigestion. Six months later, he was sixty pounds thinner and felt "springy." Ten years later he set a world weight-lifting record—and all because he analyzed his eating habits and changed them.

Horace Fletcher made this simple discovery: gulping meals made him sick and weak. He renewed his health and stamina by developing and following four basic rules: first and most important, chew your food to a pulp—at least thirty chomps per mouthful; eat only when hungry; enjoy and slowly savor the meal; never eat when emotionally or physically distressed and refuse to consider unpleasant things while eating. Scientists agree that negative emotions impair the digestion.

INSOMNIA

Lay your weary head upon a pillow stuffed with bran—that's what the Chinese did to bring on drowsiness. Or use the American frontier pillow cure of sleeping with several cushions under the head to keep an excess of blood from the brain. Or recline in the fashion of George III who, when given to fits of nervous insomnia, rested his royal head upon a pillow loosely stuffed with hops and sprinkled with alcohol, which makes the soporific effect of the hop cones even stronger. The Meskwaki Indians used hops pillows for insomnia too. Modern herbalists recommend "sleep pillows" of bruised marjoram.

A cup of hot milk should help you fall

asleep not only because it makes you feel cozy, warm, and secure like a child but also because, as the National Institute of Mental Health has pointed out, hot milk contains the amino acid tryptophan, which has a sedating effect.

Drink teas made from the sedating and relaxing herbs such as basil, marjoram, oregano, and camomile. The Italians especially rely on camomile and are known to drink it in bars as a nightcap to ensure slumber.

Whether you take hot milk or tea, always sweeten it with honey, which folk medicine maintains can help you sleep. You may also take a spoonful of honey by itself.

Attempt massaging yourself to sleep with Chinese acupressure. With your thumb, press on the center of the bottom of your heels.

Eating raw onions before retiring is an effective old English cure for insomnia, but it is best taken when sleeping alone.

"Sleeping pills" that are safe and natural are tablets of the B vitamin inositol. Dr. Atkins says that 2,000 mg. of inositol is "a remarkable sleeping medication." Calcium supplements are also said to help.

Go to bed with your head pointed north. According to the theories of yoga, that will put you in line with the flow of electromagnetic energies between the North and South poles and will thus make it easier to fall asleep. Charles Darwin believed this and followed it as a rule.

Also sleep on your right side, with your right hand under your head and your knees pulled up in the fetal position. This position takes the pressure off your heart, is said to have subtle psychic benefits, and is the position in which Buddha reclined.

KIDNEY AND BLADDER AILMENTS

Eat and drink freely of parsley. The green healer is a balm for infections of the bladder and irritation of the genitourinary tract. Richard Lucas and numerous other natural medicine experts recommend the simple parsley cure for cystitis and urinary infections. In Dutch folk medicine parsley is the main treatment for urinary problems, while an old Greek saying refers to parsley as "salvation to women," probably because of its beneficial action on cystitis. Drink parsley juice, parsley tea, and parsley based soups.

From their maize the American Indians discovered this enduring remedy for cystitis and urinary infections: corn silk tea. Corn silk is a powerful diuretic with no known side effects. The silk should be gathered before it turns brown, while the

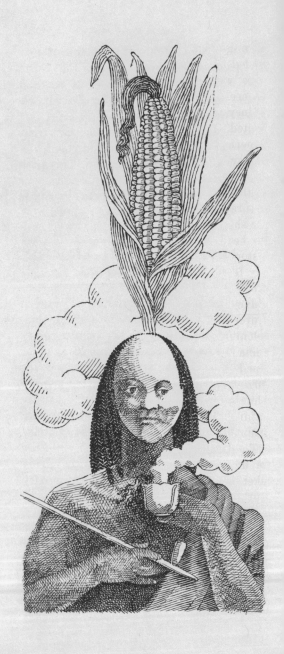

80.

corn is still very young, then steeped in boiled water. Strain and drink. This Indian cure worked so well that it became the pioneers' main ally against all bladder and kidney complaints. Corn silk tea is now accepted by the modern herbal traditions of America and Europe as a remedy for urinary tract infections.

If there is anything to the doctrine of signatures, which holds that something about the shape or character of a plant indicates its healing properties, there should be a history of the kidney bean plant as a remedy for kidney and urinary problems. And there is. The kidney pod, rather than the kidney bean itself, has been used as a diuretic in American herbal medicine from colonial times to the present. One Cincinnati doctor of years past called the combined decoction of kidney bean pods and corn silk his "most effective diuretic," while contemporary experimenters with natural healing say that the pod works amazingly well in treating urine retention.

The pods without the bean are simmered for a few hours, then the strained tea is taken throughout the day. After twenty-four hours, though, the tea loses its potency, so you must make a new pot daily.

The Cherokee Indians forbid milk to people with urinary problems. And modern Canadian doctors have found that milk can cause urinary infections in children. So it might be wise to exclude milk and milk products from your diet while sick and to cut down on them permanently if you have a tendency to get urinary tract infections.

Onion eating may help urinary weakness because onions are said to be powerfully diuretic and to cleanse the system of urea and sodium.

Pure cranberry juice or fresh cranberries are the favorite contemporary remedy of American women for cystitis. Cranberry juice contains a natural antibiotic that seems to have a most salutary effect on inflamed bladders.

The Mongolian home remedy for cystitis is a teaspoon of watermelon seed tea. Two tablespoons of the bruised seeds boiled for five minutes in a pint of water, taken a few times a day, is said to clean the bladder and kidneys. Watermelon seed tea is strongly diuretic, and South American Indians use it to reduce edema and high blood pressure.

Watermelon seeds are not advised for men, however, because their use can, it is said, cause pressure on the prostate gland. Men with urinary infections should use pumpkin seeds instead, as prescribed by American folk healers to promote the flow of urine and clean the urinary tract. And pumpkin seeds are good for the prostate.

Modern nature cures for cystitis emphasize the critical importance of extreme cleanliness in sexual encounters and toilet seat procedures. Also, urinate directly after in-

tercourse; doctors say this measure can
prevent some types of cystitis.

Many a frustrating case of honeymoon
cystitis has been soothed by a long soak in
a warm bath to which the contents of a
small box of baking soda has been added.

KIDNEY STONES

The famous seventeenth-century English
herbalist Culpeper urged the consumption
of chick-peas. Besides promoting the flow
of urine and increasing the production of
sperm, he said, "they have a cleansing
faculty, whereby they break the stone in
the kidney." His recipe was to boil them
in water until they produce a "cream,"
which should then be drunk.

It might be wise to consume fresh strawberries too. Strawberries have been prescribed by two centuries of American folk
healers in the belief that they prevent the
formation of kidney stones. As the good
Dr. Boteler said of this wonderful fruit,
"Doubtless God Almighty could have made
a better berry, but he never did."

And take grapes. American pharmacist and
herbalist Ben Charles Harris says they
eliminate acid from the system, "thus im-
mensely benefiting kidney function." A
brief mono-diet of grapes, he says, will help
eliminate gravel and stones from the kidneys and bladder (see page 38).

LARYNGITIS

Simmer raisins in water and eat the resulting raisin soup. The Tibetans say it will cure hoarseness and laryngitis, and the Arabs agree.

LEG CRAMPS, STIFFNESS, AND SWELLING

To avoid getting leg cramps, take vitamin E, vitamin B_6, vitamin C, and calcium supplements. When you get leg cramps at night, lie on your back and flex (do not point) your feet, pulling your toes and feet toward your shins.

To prevent your legs from getting stiff, a spry 106-year-old Henry Jones recommended rubbing the back of them with a slice of lemon.

LOSS OF WEIGHT AND LACK OF APPETITE

The folk healers of India and China maintain that fresh ginger always stimulates the appetite. Chew it by itself or with some rock salt.

India Ayurvedic doctors also prescribe the following slightly more elaborate remedy to arouse the desire to eat: a tonic compounded from fresh ginger, black grape juice, cardamom, cinnamon, cloves, and pepper, two to four teaspoons taken before meals. When taken after eating, this tonic improves digestion, they say. Additional benefits are that it will also "remove constipation, bring sound sleep, allay fatigue and supply energy and charm in life."

People afflicted with extreme weight loss might try adorning themselves with emeralds, for according to gem therapy the emerald's cosmic rays have "a distinctly fattening effect." Not only that, emeralds are supposed to help cure syphilis, headaches, ulcers, influenza, poor digestion, idleness, and the tendency to show off. According to the ancient Egyptians, emeralds also improve eyesight.

LIVER AND GALL-BLADDER DISORDERS

The supreme aid for ailing livers is the humble, hearty dandelion. Dandelion roots and stems have been a major hepatic medicine throughout centuries, used with veneration by Europeans and Asiatics of wise repute. In the seventeenth century Culpeper called the dandelion "very effective for the obstructions of the liver, gallbladder, and spleen, and the diseases that arise from them, . . ." then went on to praise Dutch and French physicians for prescribing it, remarking that such doctors are "not so selfish as ours are, but more communicative of the virtues of plants to people." Both observations still hold true.

Dandelion is still the liver's good friend for two reasons, according to modern herbalist John Lust: it promotes the formation of bile and it removes excess water from the body in edemous conditions resulting from liver problems. But people don't know its virtues and the innocent little dandelion is slaughtered regularly every spring and summer across the lawns of America. Gather dandelions whenever you can. Take a decoction of the roots in white wine, the leaves in salads and soups, leaves, and/or roots as tea and, most effective, fresh juice.

A very basic and helpful remedy for a sluggish liver prescribed by Welsh and American grannies is lemon juice added to hot boiled water. This should be taken first thing in the morning.

An old Cuban remedy for jaundice demands olfactory stamina and considerable faith. For thirteen days you must wear thirteen cloves of garlic strung around your neck. On the thirteenth night, proceed to a corner where two streets meet, take off your necklace, and fling it behind you while running away without looking back to see where it lands.

The best solid food to start the gallbladder working is said to be bran—organic, raw bran, not the commercial cereal variety. Have it for breakfast—do not skip breakfast if you have a faulty gallbladder. Bran is a high-fiber food, and English physicians have stated that a high-fiber diet "sweeps the degenerated bile salt out of the colon," improving the gallbladder conditions of many people who try it.

The Taoists believe that radish juice is a great benefit to the liver. The Japanese and Tibetans believe that radishes eaten raw benefit the liver greatly. The Russians believe that the greatest liver benefit is their black radish. All around, it seems wise to eat radishes if you're feeling "liverish."

Naturopaths say that those with faulty livers should consume quantities of the following: carrots, artichokes, asparagus, spinach, chicory, watercress, parsley, chervil, apples, strawberries, grapes, and drink teas of rosemary, marjoram, mint, camomile, and, especially, sage. "Sage boiled in wine and water purifies the liver and kidney," said Father Kneipp, renowned nineteenth-century German priest-healer.

For gallbladder problems Mexicans brew a small piece of artichoke leaf into a tea and drink it every morning.

For all disorders of the liver and spleen the Chinese rely on red rose petals, eaten fresh or made into a tea (see page 68).

MALE COMPLAINTS

Since one out of every four American men over fifty-two years of age is reportedly afflicted with prostate disorders, American men might be wise to start munching pumpkin seeds regularly. Hungarian gypsies, Bulgarian mountain men, and Transylvanian Germans have long used pumpkin seeds to preserve the prostate.

No one knows exactly why pumpkin seeds work so well on the prostate, but some conjecture it's because the seeds contain nutrients—B vitamins, phosphorus, iron, and zinc—that are essential for reproductive function. The prostate contains ten times more zinc than most other organs in the body.

Oysters contain a remarkably high content of zinc, so their beneficial effect on the prostate may account for their reputation as potent aphrodisiacs.

For seminal weakness or spermatorrhea, the Ayurvedic master Dastur says a cure can be effected by three days of eating saffron well soaked in clarified butter. Or one and a half ounces of the flour of kidney beans cooked with milk and served hot with a bit of clarified butter.

If you're not inclined to have saffron or kidney beans, how about oatmeal or rolled oats? Modern herbalist Joseph Kadams reports oat eating helps control this problem.

To treat the problem of premature ejaculation, use Japanese shiatsu along the spine in the sacrum area—from the coccyx to the bottom of the small of the back. Press each point lightly for three seconds ten times. Also press the pit of the stomach (beneath the breastbone) with three fingers ten times, five seconds each time. Shiatsu master Tokujiro Namikoshi proclaims that this exercise will "assist men of more than fifty years of age in performing the sexual act several times with only one ejaculation: loss of large amounts of sperm is fatiguing."

A natural contraceptive for men may be raw cottonseed oil, according to the modern Chinese. In the 1950's they discovered that men were becoming sterile in communes where this cooking oil was used extensively in food preparation. In the 1970's the Chinese isolated gossypol, the oil's anti-fertility agent, which, they report, has proved 99.9 percent effective in killing sperm or drastically reducing sperm count.

MEMORY LOSS
AND MENTAL FATIGUE

That rosemary's for remembrance we cannot forget. Shakespeare immortalized the association, but it has prevailed since Grecian times when students took rosemary to aid their powers of recall before examina-

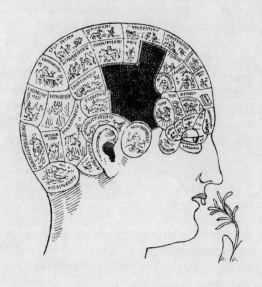

tions. The Italians, Arabs, and Chinese also believe it strengthens the memory. In addition to drinking rosemary tea, you can wear or eat essential oil of rosemary for the same results. Apply it to the vertebrae in the neck.

Back in 1597 barber-surgeon-botanist Gerard wrote that sage "quickeneth the senses and memory." Contemporary holistic herbalists say that sage's action is beneficial in combating mental exhaustion and that it strengthens the ability to concentrate. In the Middle Ages, infusions of sage in mulled wine were provided to restore youthful powers to the aged. Whether in wine or as tea, take sage often to regain powers of mind.

In the West Indies, the medicine men make teas from fresh ginger and cloves to overcome sluggish thinking and quicken the senses. Other herbs with reputations for heightening mental powers are fennel, chervil, and according to the Taoists, tarragon.

To refresh the brain and enhance its powers, learn and practice the half-headstand, a simple yoga technique. It stimulates the brain by supplying it with rich, oxygenated blood. It also stimulates the pituitary and pineal glands, strengthens the memory, and improves the ability to concentrate.

Sit on the floor with your calves tucked under your thighs Japanese style. Cross your arms and grasp your elbows with the opposite hands. Bend over and place elbows and forearms on the floor in front of you. Keeping elbows where they are placed, interlace your fingers so that you've formed a triangle with your elbows and intermeshed hands. Place the back of your head inside your cupped palms, with the top of your head to the ground. Tucking your toes underneath your feet, straighten your legs and push your behind up in the air so that your body is now shaped like a "mountain." You will feel the blood rushing to your head. Hold for a minute or so, and with practice build up to five minutes and longer. Then come down out of the posture and remain quiet and relaxed for a few moments. Eventually you may be able to ''walk up'' into a full headstand. Caution: people with high or low blood pressure should not attempt headstands.

MOTION SICKNESS

The *Barefoot Doctor's Manual* of present-day China explains that motion sickness is primarily due to a dysfunction of the vestibular nerve that maintains the body's equilibrium. To prevent this sickness, the manual says, one should keep one's eyes on some distant, nonmoving object. Do not close your eyes. Should the illness occur, use the tip of·your thumb and the side of your index finger to ''pinch and pull'' the flesh in the center, inner side of your wrist about an inch below your hand. Doing this before starting a trip will help prevent motion sickness.

In Mexico, wise people who have to travel in crowded buses over bumpy roads put a copper penny in the navel to prevent motion sickness.

An American home remedy is to consume a well-beaten mixture of egg whites and lemon juice just before traveling or to suck a lemon as soon as the feeling of motion sickness begins.

NAUSEA AND VOMITING

Hippocrates prescribed mint to end vomiting, and his advice is still followed around the world. Chewed fresh or as tea, antiseptic mint is said to end vomiting and act as a balm to the entire digestive tract. Even its aroma can quell feelings of sickness. Mint has many virtues and tastes divine. As the old herbalist Gerard wrote, "The smell rejoiceth the heart of man"; it also repels rats.

An equally well-known antidote for queasiness is ginger. It is especially beloved by the Chinese, who valued it as a quieter of nausea, "corrector of fetor," and conqueror of mushroom poisoning. Eat it raw or drink it as a tea or diluted juice.

The nausea caused by radiation and chemotherapy treatments for cancer may be greatly alleviated by marijuana, according to medical evidence.

Babies who are spitting up can be given the contemporary American home cure: a little heavy syrup from canned peaches. Nauseated adults may benefit from room temperature Coca-Cola.

NERVOUSNESS, DEPRESSION, AND DISORDERS OF THE PSYCHE

Marjoram has been said to calm all grief, "even the pangs of love." Some witty healers prescribe pizza for a broken heart, since oregano is a slightly stronger form of marjoram. A pinch of marjoram or oregano will help vanquish nervous tics, and a glass of marjoram tea has a pronounced tranquilizing effect in depression. As Gerard wrote, "it easeth such as are given to overmuch sighing." Be warned, however, that too much marjoram is stupefying.

The Elizabethans were fond of the peaceful feeling brought on by the sweet little camomile flower. The apple-scented blossom's reputation as a pacifier of agitated and despondent minds is still very strong in most of Europe, especially Italy and Greece, and here in America. If only they'd serve it in psychiatric hospitals instead of endless cups of jittery-making coffee . . .

Other psychiatric spice-rack cures widely recommended for nervousness, depression, and hysterical disorders are basil, rosemary, sage, clove, and thyme.

Melancholics should make love. According to the ancient medical traditions of Tibet and Persia, sexual intercourse can help

overcome feelings of depression and melancholy, especially for people who are obsessed with the longing for sex.

Nature healers prescribe the juice of
equal amounts of watercress and spinach to
wash away the blues. Carrot, apple, celery,
and orange juice also have a cheering effect
and overcome nervousness.

And do watch what you wear. According
to color therapy, pinks and scarlets are a
boon for withdrawn depressives and cata-
tonics. Nervous, high-strung people, however, must not wear pink or live in pink
houses as the exciting bright tones are
likely to drive them over the edge. Give
them blues and violets instead.

Yellowy oranges cheer everyone up, and
good old green, the color of nature, is
known to have an overall harmonizing effect.

Try the age-old remedy of a long soak in
a warm bath; it is calming and sedative.
Enhance its effect by adding a strong solution made from camomile or lavender flowers. Or add a few drops of essential oil of
rose, jasmine, lavender, or sandalwood to
the tub. All of these have been prescribed
for anxiety and depression.

Quilt lavender flowers into a cap and
wear it daily to "comfort the braine," as
suggested by William Turner in 1551.
Lavender is traditionally said to be espe-

cially good for all kinds of mental disorders
—depression, hysteria, panic, palpitations,
delusions, hysterical paralysis, irritability,
apoplexy, convulsions, and "the tremblings
and passions of the heart." Besides putting
lavender in your hat, also put some in your
bath, take two spoonfuls of distilled water
of lavender flowers, drink lavender tea, apply the perfume to the temples and nostrils,
or simply sniff the lovely fragrance for its
calming effect.

For nervous tremors, palsy, and trembling
of the limbs, drink sage tea. John Wesley
claimed that it kept his hand as steady as
that of a fifteen-year-old. Also apply the
leaves "sodden in wine" to the affected
places.

In terms of edibles, lean heavily on apples,
an old European cure for melancholy,
nervousness, and insomnia, and on celery,
prescribed by Hippocrates and the Chinese
for nervous hysterics. Of celery, an American folk healer once said, "No medicine is
really so efficacious in cases of nervous
prostration," adding that onions were the
next best bet. And stay away from refined
sugars and junk food. They send your
spirits soaring, but they quickly burn out,
dropping you suddenly into a devastating,
depressing crash.

All depressed, nervous, and frazzled people
should be reminded to take their vitamins,
particularly the B complex and especially

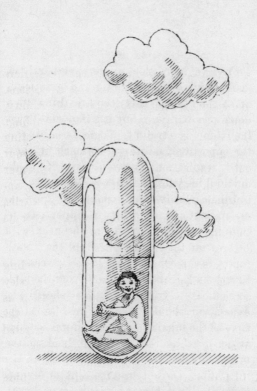

B_1, B_2, and folic acid. Vitamin B_3 (niacin) has been used successfully in orthomolecular psychiatry to treat schizophrenia.

To release physical and mental tension, try yoga's "corpse pose": Lie on your back, legs spread slightly and arms slightly out from the side of the body, palms facing upward. Remain this way for five to ten minutes. Completely let go of your muscles; let the floor support you. Give yourself the positive suggestion to relax; imagine all the tension melting out of you. Just rest this way and enjoy it.

To relieve depression, anxiety, and fatigue, learn yogic deep breathing and practice it often. You can do this deep breathing lying down or sitting up, but it's important that the spine is straight. Yogic breathing is the opposite of military "stomach in, chest out" respiration. Instead, it is deep, abdominal breathing.

Inhale slowly and expand the gut (do not suck it in), then fill the upper part of the chest all the way up to the neck with the rest of the inhalation. Hold the breath for a few seconds, then *slowly* release it, first from the abdomen, then from the midsection, then from the upper chest. The exhalation should take at least as much time as the inhalation, and preferably twice as long, while the period of holding the breath should be at least as long as the inhalation. Do not breathe fast or hyperventilate. Just breathe deeply and slowly, concentrating on receiving positive energy with the in-breath and on releasing tension or anxiety with the out-breath. After ten to twenty of these complete breaths, sit quietly for a few moments, eyes closed, breathing normally, and feeling at peace.

Yogic breathing circulates the revitalizing *prana*, or life energy, throughout the body. It oxygenates the blood sent to the brain, thereby increasing memory span and learning capacity. It is said to be helpful in fighting all disease, especially when combined with visualization and positive suggestion. Since you have to breathe every moment of your life, you might as well learn to do it to optimum effect.

Dr. Edward Bach, a British physician and biochemist of this century, developed a system of self-healing based on the idea that the mind's negative emotions create illness and that certain flowers have the power to alter these emotions. Bach's flower remedies, which treat the patient's personality rather than the disease, are categorized according to basic temperaments and anxieties. Among the thirty-eight flower remedies Dr. Bach discovered are chicory for self-pity, clematis for indifference, gentian for doubt, impatiens for tension, mustard for melancholia, olive for mental fatigue, pine for guilt, rock rose for terror, and sweet chestnut for suicidal depression. You can make them yourself with a little effort.

Fill a clean glass bowl with spring water and add freshly picked flower heads until they completely cover the surface of the water. This is best done right in the field where the blossoms are plucked. Let stand in the hot sun for four hours. Then lift out flowers with a few blades of grass or straw and transfer the "potenized" water into a small vial. Fill halfway, then add good brandy until full (it preserves the solution). Take these flower tinctures often; you only need a few drops.

Dr. Bach's theories scandalized the medical profession, but patients flocked to him and even other doctors reported amazing success with his remedies. Since Dr. Bach considered good health a birthright of humanity, he never charged for his services.

NIGHTMARES

Nightmares, pain, insomnia, and excess of sexual desire may all be quelled by a little lettuce. The latex that oozes from the wounded plant—most powerful in lettuce that has gone to seed—is sedative, narcotic, and anesthetic. The dried latex is sometimes called "lettuce opium." Besides taking the edge off anxiety, frustration, and carnal lust—the reason Pythagoras called it the "plant of eunuchs"—lettuce brings pleasant visions and sweet dreams. The sooner it is eaten after being picked, the stronger the results. Eat the leaves or take a tea of them before going to bed.

A thirteenth-century Arab manuscript says of rosemary: "If the leaves be put beneath your pillow, you will be protected from troublesome dreams and all mental anxiety." According to European herbal lore, if you put daisy roots under your pillow, you will have sweet dreams of the one you love.

Other handy preventives against the onslaught of demon dreams are cabbage water (brewed with a bit of sage), thyme, catnip, peppermint, or anise, the last being the favorite of the ancient Greeks.

NOSEBLEEDS

American grandmother methods include putting your feet in hot water to draw the blood from the head; raising your arm on the same side as the bloody nostril; and placing a dime on the roof of the mouth and holding it there with the tongue until the bleeding stops.

Use Japanese finger pressure therapy on the medulla oblongata (at the base of the skull in the top back of the neck). Tilt the head back and with your right thumb apply pressure until the bleeding stops.

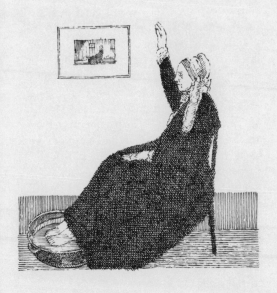

Another finger pressure technique comes from modern medicine: The nose should be squeezed with the thumb and forefinger just below its hard portion. The pressure should be maintained for at least five minutes, say Drs. Vickery and Fries.

The Red Cross says to put the head back (do not lie down) and apply cold compresses or ice to the bridge of the nose. Nature healers say the ice should be applied to the back of the neck.

OBESITY AND THYROID DISORDERS

Learn the shoulder stand. All manner of swamis, yogis, and maharishis say it is simply supreme for overall good health. In particular, it is excellent for the thyroid gland. The position massages and stimulates it, thereby toning up the whole metabolism and giving you added energy.

Lie flat on your back, raise your legs and hips off the ground until you are "standing on your shoulders." Keep your upper arms and elbows on the floor and support your back with your hands. You will feel the pressure on your throat.

Even obese people can do a modified shoulder stand: lie on the floor, knees tucked up toward the chest and buttocks just a few inches from a wall. Put feet up on the wall and straighten legs, pushing the trunk up off the floor and putting pressure on the neck.

Retain the position for one to twenty minutes. Come out of it slowly, rolling the back down, then lowering the legs, all the while keeping your head on the floor.

New York nutritionist and chiropractor Jairo Rodriguez offers this cure for obesity. But be careful: it can be harmful if taken in excess. *Mix one drop only* of a two percent iodine solution into twenty-four ounces of plain water. Each day drink eight ounces of the mixture, but *never more* than that. Iodine stimulates the thyroid and is converted to thyroxine, which breaks down fats and normalizes metabolism.

If you follow this prescription exactly, says Rodriguez, you will see dramatic results in weight loss. But take heed once again: iodine is corrosive to the tissues. Too much will not make you thinner, it will make you sick—you may break out or experience a burning sensation in the throat and chest. If that happens, the antidote is to eat bread and crackers, since starch neutralizes the effects of iodine poisoning. This treatment should only be done under the supervision of a medical professional. An absolutely safe way of consuming iodine is to eat lots of iodine-rich foods from the ocean—like sea salt, seaweed, and fish.

Less dangerous than iodine (but more expensive) is the jewel cure. For it you need a moonstone or a topaz. These gems, when viewed through a prism, are seen to give off blue rays. These "cosmic blue rays," explains Indian jewel therapist Battacharaya, regulate the metabolism and also control the fat system and endocrine glands.

Besides getting you thinner, he says, moonstones and topazes may cure you of laryngitis, goiter, chicken pox, palpitations, toothache, hypocrisy, fondness for lawsuits, talkativeness, insanity, and feelings of self-importance.

According to a turn-of-the-century American physician, "insatiable hunger and canine appetite" are often cured by applying a small bit of bread dipped in wine to the nostrils.

Natural health expert Carlson Wade says it helps to drink lots of hot liquids because they make you feel full (boiled water has no calories); other nature healers assure us that apples and cherries benefit the dieter.

A teaspoon of honey before meals is recommended for dieters in India and Pakistan. The honey will dampen your appetite, they say, as well as satisfy your craving for sweets. Raw-juice therapists also recommend a teaspoon of honey before meals for people on diets.

SEXUAL ENNUI, IMPOTENCE, AND FRIGIDITY

A languid libido may be pepped up with mint. Legend has it that the mint plant was originally a beautiful nymph named Menthe. So desirable was Menthe that the god Pluto fell in love with her, exciting such jealousy in his wife, Proserpina, that she trampled Menthe into the ground. But the nymph came back as the herb mint with the power to excite sexual desire in whoever eats it.

Mint is widely known as an aphrodisiac among the French, the Arabs, and the English, who mix their mint with vinegar to stir up venery and bodily lust. And the Queen of Sheba, a woman most renowned for her sexual stamina, consumed a daily love potion made from crushed mint mixed with carrot, potato, and cabbage juices.

The Bambara of Mali, Africa, deal with impotence this way: take the bark from an old tamarind tree, mix with salt, and pulverize. Add the powder to a soup made from the testicles of a ram and the kidneys of an old rooster. Eat this in the evening.

Although their scents are hardly the essence of romance, onions and garlic are widely credited with arousing sexual desire and increasing sexual ability. The

Hindus prescribe white onion juice for loss of virility, preferably mixed with fresh ginger and honey; take it daily for three weeks. Certain Frenchmen ascribe their ability to make love day and night to a steady diet of garlic, and Henry IV is said to have owed his erotic prowess to the potent bulb.

Other foods with reputations as aphrodisiacs are celery, asparagus (because of its similarity to the phallus), chicken eggs, peaches (whose juice symbolizes, to the Chinese, feminine love libations), chestnuts, oysters (Casanova sometimes had fifty of them for breakfast and called them "a spur to the spirit and to love"), and truffles (a favorite of Mme. Pompadour and supposed cause of Napoleon's ability to sire a son).

Ginseng and honey also have a long noble history in this libidinous regard. The Chinese and American Indians both used ginseng as an aphrodisiac (ginseng is native to America and used to be exported to China), while honey's power to increase sexual energy has been put forth by Galen, Ovid, and Sheikh Nefzawi, author of Islam's pillow book, *The Perfumed Garden*.

Licorice, which contains measurable amounts of female hormones, is a favorite aphrodisiac of the Hindus and is prescribed in their ancient love manual, the *Kāmasūtra*. Mix it with equal amounts of milk and honey to produce a "nectar-like composition . . . provocative of sexual vigor." The French use it as an aphrodisiac, too. They mix a teaspoon of the powdered root in a glass of plain soda water.

Other spices and herbs said to overcome impotence, frigidity, and lack of lust are anise, basil, fennel, fenugreek, cinnamon, ginger, nutmeg, pepper, caraway, coriander, rosemary, and thyme. And we should mention sesame seeds. In ancient Babylon, women ate halvah, which is made of sesame seeds and honey, to restore their sex appeal and drive. Nutritionist and author Paavo Airola reports that sesame seeds are rich in magnesium and potassium, while honey is rich in aspartic acid, all of which have been used to treat the "tired housewife syndrome."

Plutarch said that "the soul of a man in love is full of perfumes and sweet odours." Turn this statement around by using sweet-smelling oils of rose and jasmine and sandalwood for their aphrodisiac effect. For all romantic liaisons use rose essence, a fragrance linked with the passion of love for incalculable ages. Rose blended with sandalwood is an ancient Hindu aphrodisiac.

To deal with cold-hearted lovers use jasmine, which is "emotionally warming" and "a giver of confidence." Five to ten drops of jasmine essence added to a hip bath will definitely bring on a mood of languor. Similarly, brews of rose and jasmine flowers are said to have a pronounced romantic effect. You can mix the flowers in with a little black tea.

Sexual responsiveness, as you no doubt know, can be heightened by careful touches, but Japanese shiatsu finger pressure therapy has this down to a science. According to shiatsu, the sexual responsiveness of both men and women is positively affected by strong pressure along the four inches of the bottom of the spine, the point in the pit of the stomach, and the points along the sides of the spine in the small of the back. Additionally, for women, pressure should be applied to the inguinal regions—on the front of the body where the thighs join the hips. Press hard.

For a jewel cure, rely on diamonds, truly a girl's best friend and here's why: Ruled by Venus, the sign of love, the indigo cosmic rays released by diamonds are supposed to help overcome fear of the opposite sex, sterility, frigidity, impotence, gonorrhea, menopause, facial paralysis, diabetes, convulsions, delirium tremens, and every conceivable obsession.

Take your vitamins—E, B_6, and folic acid. They're said to keep the sex glands healthy and to arouse desire. Folic acid has been dubbed "frolic acid" because of its ability to bring out the sex drive in otherwise romantically depressed alcoholics. As for

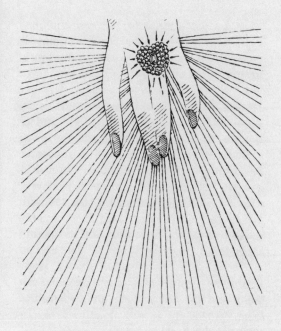

vitamin E and B$_6$, nutritionist Adelle Davis said they are "essential" for a hot and healthy reproductive system.

SINUS TROUBLES

Teas of fenugreek and golden seal are strongly recommended for sinus problems and for all inflammations of the mucous membranes with excessive secretion and discharge. Garlic tea may also relieve sinus inflammations. Steep two to four cloves of freshly chopped garlic in a quart of boiling water. Strain and drink one to four cups a day.

Rely on eucalyptus or peppermint oils, both of which are said to be antiseptic, expectorant, and antispasmodic and ever so useful in respiratory disorders. If you don't have the bottled essences, you can release the oil by crushing the leaves of the plants. Drop in boiling water and inhale the steam; massage oil onto the congested area, or rub it into the reflex points on the feet that control the sinuses.

Rub the underside tips of the toes. According to foot reflexology these spots are the reflex points for the sinuses, and massaging them will help relieve inflamed sinuses.

Drain the sinuses with the yoga cleansing technique of *neti*. Yogis do an extreme form of this by threading a long string through the nasal passages, but you don't have to go that far. Instead, use room temperature water (bottled, boiled, or distilled is preferred) and suck it up through your nose. Expel the water through the mouth. It may sting a little, especially if the congestion and inflammation are acute, but it will clear your sinuses and head. Avoid blowing the nose hard afterward; that is always bad for the sinuses. Regular practice of *neti*, it is said, "bestows sharp eyesight and soon destroys the multitude of diseases above the shoulder region."

Eat horseradish. This stimulating condiment, used as a medicine since the Middle Ages, is a popular remedy for numerous ailments, including sinus problems. A mixture of grated horseradish and lemon juice taken by the half-teaspoonful between meals may smart a bit but is said to clear the mucus of chronic sinus inflammations when taken for a few months.

Classically used to treat dropsy, kidney conditions, and languid digestion, the gypsies use it to cure colds and coughs.

SKIN PROBLEMS

Try pampering your complexion with urine. It may sound repulsive, but this method has a history of good results. In the American South in the eighteenth and nineteenth centuries, both whites and blacks attributed their clear, smooth skin to daily urine treatments. The fastidious Pennsylvania Germans and the earthier peasants of the Sierra Madres all used urine washes to make the skin "handsome" and clear up acne. In Spain they used it to remove freckles, as well as to brush the teeth.

In Texas, a remedy for acne is to wash your face with a baby's wet diaper—good advice since the preferred urine to use is that of a child who has not yet absorbed the pollutants of civilization. Additionally, the best urine medicine is that taken from a healthy person's first passing in the morning.

Urine is especially good at fighting staph infections and will clear up psoriasis, some

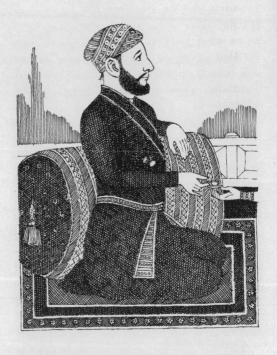

say, if drunk as well as applied locally.

Drink urine? When he was in his eighties, India's ex-Prime Minister Desai confounded the modern world by explaining that he attributed his health and stamina to the fact that he drank a glass of his own urine every day. Maurice Wilson, who made a solo attempt on Mount Everest, also attributed his strength to urine fasts and washes. Urine has been extensively used as medicine in India and is prescribed in ancient Ayurvedic texts.

It has been claimed that in addition to maintaining general good health, urine drinking can actually cure gangrene, jaundice, and cancer. Recently, Danish scientists have extracted a substance from urine which reportedly allays anxiety better than chemical tranquilizers and has no side effects. Further, investigative health journalist Gary Null reports that a new experimental anticancer treatment has been developed from the antineoplastons extracted from urine.

So if you're ready for a new adventure in health, start drinking your own urine in the morning after you first relieve your bladder. Let a little urine pass, then catch a half cup of the midflow; empty the rest of your bladder as usual.

Baths may be esthetically more pleasing than urine washes. Itchy skin can be relieved by oatmeal or cornstarch baths. For the latter, follow these directions from Florida naturopath Samuel Homola. Mix a pound of cornstarch with cold water to make a paste, then add hot water and boil the mixture till it's thick; add result to tub of warm water. Soak for fifteen minutes. Pat yourself dry, leaving a slight film on your skin.

Baking soda, two tablespoons or more to the tub, also relieves the itching, as do sage baths. The French say thyme baths will soothe a host of skin disorders. Add a large sprig of thyme or some thyme tea to the daily bath. Thyme contains the antiseptic, antibacterial substance thymol.

Taking 10,000 units of vitamin A daily is said to combat dry skin, from 400 to 800 units of vitamin E a day along with B complex to fight eczema, and B$_6$ to control acne and psoriasis.

For psoriasis, water therapists suggest daubing the scaly patches with real seawater or with water that has been saturated with sea salt. Get thyself to the seaside and dip often in the surf.

To remove acne scars, advises herbalist Dian Buchman, apply a teaspoon of powdered nutmeg and honey, or nutmeg and vitamin E oil. Allow to dry on the skin for twenty minutes. Apply once a week. Also, rub vitamin E on stretch marks and scars to speed healing.

For divine facials, use natural substances from the kitchen, such as yogurt or papaya. After eating a papaya, save its skin and rub the inside of it on your clean face and neck. It will dry to a translucent mask. Leave on for ten to twenty minutes, during which time the papaya enzyme papain will be hard at work removing dead skin cells and freckles. When you wash it off with warm water, you'll be surprised at how smooth and radiant your complexion is and how much tighter the pores are.

Similarly, slices of strawberries and cucumbers can be rubbed onto the face to lighten and refresh the complexion. Ukrainian girls pat whole-milk yogurt or sour cream onto their faces to restore elasticity and rejuvenate the skin. A mask of honey imparts a healthy glow to the complexion and is really marvelous for dry skin. Lemon juice tightens and lightens the skin; the Polynesians use it mixed with rose water to remove freckles.

Most Americans are unaware of the healing heritage of golden seal, a native plant with near-miraculous properties. The yellowish golden seal root was one of the favorite remedies of the American Indians, who introduced it to the pioneers, the settlers, and eventually the international world of herbal medicine. A tea made from the root, applied externally, seems to excel in the treatment of skin diseases and inflammations such as open sores, erysipelas, acne, eczema, and ringworm. Use carefully since it stains. Dab on as a wash, cleanse with hydrogen peroxide, then sprinkle on the powdered root and cover. The tea taken internally at the same time is said to enhance the effectiveness.

Golden seal tea has been used by the Indians for a variety of ailments, from inflammations of the mucous membranes to colds, flu, general weakness, stomach and liver troubles, morning sickness (in small, frequent doses), poor circulation, bowel, bladder and prostate troubles, indigestion, sore mouth and gums, weak eyes, VD, hemorrhoids, and nausea.

For tea or wash, steep one teaspoon of the powdered root in a pint of boiling hot water, stir, let cool and settle, pour off liquid, and take one tablespoon of it four to six times a day or take it in capsule form.

An African tribal cure for ringworm is a paste of papaya applied to the affected skin.

To heal eczema and other skin conditions, herbalist Alma Hutchens says an external wash with strong strawberry leaves is extremely effective.

SPRAINS AND SWELLINGS

The advice of the Red Cross is to keep the sprained limb elevated. Water therapists and naturopaths advise applying a cold fomentation or ice pack immediately after getting the sprain.

The Afro-American and European remedy is to apply red or blue clay taken from a creek or any muddy place, according to Hoodoo medicine historian Faith Mitchell. The clay may be applied alone or mixed with vinegar.

Another Afro-American cure is to cut off the top of a toadstool, dry it, dampen it with whisky, and then apply it to the problem area. Afro-Americans, American Indians, and Europeans agree on the mullein cure for sprains and swellings (see page 12).

TOOTH, GUM, MOUTH, AND THROAT PROBLEMS

Wiggle your toothbrush bristles to fight decay and degeneration of the teeth and gums. This method of brushing developed by Dr. Bass, dean emeritus of Tulane University School of Medicine in Louisiana, is so effective that even your dentist will tell you to do it. Put a soft, thin-bristled brush at a forty-five-degree angle into the crevice where the gums meet the teeth. Pressing down firmly, vibrate it there to massage the gums, which may bleed at first, and to dislodge the plaque. Finish off the area by firmly drawing the brush over the surface of the tooth toward its tip. And better than toothpaste, brush with baking soda and a drop or two of hydrogen peroxide. New research reveals that this potent mixture kills the germs and bacteria that cause degeneration of the gums.

Food for teeth: Alfalfa sprouts rebuild decayed choppers, reports Dr. H. E. Kirschner, a foremost admirer of "nature's healing grasses." Eating strawberries gets rid of tooth discoloration and removes tartar, say the homeopaths. Furthermore, according to the French, apples whiten the teeth, massage the gums, and disinfect the mouth.

For toothache, sore gums, and mouth ulcers, boil the roots of your geranium plants and use the solution for a mouth wash as the Meskwaki Indians did. Spit out. Or use the Alabama Indians' favorite remedy —insert the root of common goldenrod into the painful cavity. The Zuni Indians chewed goldenrod blossoms to cure a sore throat.

Sage saves once again. According to Chinese and American folk medicine, sage makes an excellent gargle for sore throats, tonsillitis, and ulcerated mouths. A hot infusion of sage tea, as a mouth rinse, is the Russian peasants' main remedy for toothache. It is also said to prevent tooth decay.

As most of us know, gargling with warm salt water helps relieve the pain of sore throats and inflamed gums.

Clove oil is a local anesthetic; it deadens the aching sensation of teeth and gums and has been used for this purpose since cloves were first brought to Europe by traders from Macao. If you don't have any clove oil, steep some bruised whole cloves in hot water or honey to mobilize the essential oil, then keep the clove in your mouth next to the painful spot.

Nineteenth-century abolitionist Lydia Child, in a book titled *The Frugal Housewife,* explained that the slimy tea of common dark blue violets (flowers and leaves) made an excellent cure for cankers. The French say blueberry eating cures cankers.

The modern vitamin remedy for canker sores and bleeding gums is lots of vitamin C.

ULCERS

To relieve gastric and peptic ulcers, drink licorice root water or suck on real licorice candy. Licorice root, underrated and practically unknown among modern Americans, was one of the main medicines of the ancients and has been venerated for its healing powers for over forty centuries. The Egyptians thought so highly of it that they stored huge quantities of it among the treasures in King Tut's tomb to refresh and revive the pharaoh in the afterlife.

According to British physician William Thompson, licorice has a cortisonelike action that facilitates the healing process. In fact, he says, carbenoxolene, a licorice derivative, is a drugstore medicine sold for gastric ulcers. Herbalist Dian Buchman reports that researchers in Japan, where licorice is a widely used folk medicine, say it can inhibit gastric secretions and would therefore help people suffering from ulcers.

For duodenal ulcers, follow the wisdom of the Chinese: eat honey. Honey is an alkaline food and it neutralizes stomach acids. The darker the honey, e.g., buckwheat honey, the higher the alkaline level. The darker honeys are also richer in minerals, especially magnesium.

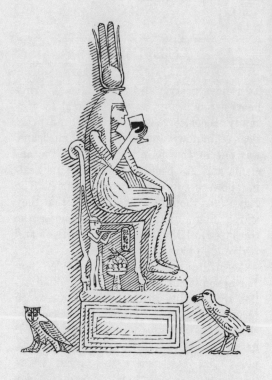

Although red pepper is hot, it is not an irritant. Red pepper is a wonderful all-purpose healer used in indigenous medical traditions around the world.

In South America, where it got its name, cayenne pepper (capsicum) is used as emergency ulcer treatment, as therapy for chronic peptic and bleeding ulcers, and for numerous other complaints. For ulcers, begin the treatment by taking one-quarter teaspoon of ground cayenne with a glass of water on an empty stomach. Increase the amount by one-quarter teaspoon daily until you get up to three tablespoons three times a day.

VARICOSE VEINS

Munch marigold flowers, a standard herbal remedy for varicose veins and circulatory problems. The fresh flower petals may be applied raw or as an ointment (made by mixing the dry, powdered petals with honey and some butter or oil). In addition, an infusion of the healing flowers (made by pouring boiling water over an ounce of the dry, powdered petals and stems) can be used as a hot foot bath and as a tea—three tablespoons of it three times a day is the recommended dosage. In this way, by using marigold inside and out, varicose veins may be banished, they say.

The cheerful flower is also said to be good for scars, sprains, cuts, eczema, depression, toothache, and leukorrhea. Henry VII took marigold in his pestilence medicine, and the gypsies have used it for centuries to clean and heal wounds.

Taking up to 1,000 units of vitamin E a day is reportedly effective against varicose veins, blood clots, and phlebitis. Try massaging the problem area with vitamin E oil or essential oil of cypress. The woody, spicy cypress oil is also, like marigolds, said to be effective when used locally on hemorrhoids.

WARTS

Gather precious wart-removing medicine from dandelion stems, as the European gypsies do. The milky juice that flows from a broken dandelion stalk, when applied to a wart, makes it disappear incredibly fast. Touch the juice to the wart and let dry. Repeat two or three times a day for a few days. Then the wart should turn dark and fall off by itself. According to all reports, this is not a gypsy con, but one of their great simple cures.

Since fresh dandelions are in season only in the spring and summer, at other times try these American folk remedies on the ugly protuberances: Rub them with a rind of bacon, or with soft green walnuts, or with a slice of raw potato, or with a radish, or with a raw onion dipped in salt (sleep with this applied to the wart for a week). Or, and this may be simplest, empty a vitamin E capsule into a Band-Aid and place that over the wart.

WEAKNESS AND FATIGUE

To pep up the aged and to stimulate the flagging energies of sickly children, baths of sage, rosemary, and/or thyme are recommended by the French. Sprigs of the herbs by themselves or equal handfuls of them,

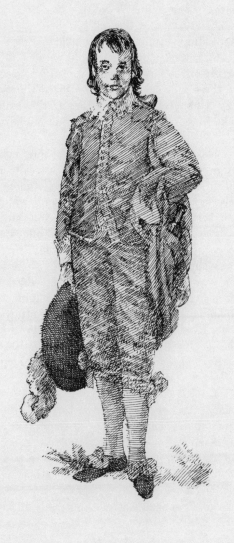

123.

placed in a linen bag or similar container for neatness' sake, are put into the tub. A similar effect can be had by taking a tea of the same pep-up herbs. Do not take these baths or teas before bedtime.

According to nineteenth-century English doctors, weak children should occasionally be given the "remarkably useful" remedy of three teaspoons of sherry three times a day. Older convalescents, they said, should take glassfuls of sherry, port, or Madeira.

To restore vigor and banish fatigue, consume iodine-rich seaweeds and sea salt, as an iodine deficiency can cause lethargy; rely on occasional doses of ginseng which has been shown to have significant anti-fatigue effects; and include the following foods in your diet which are recommended by naturopaths as energy boosters: pumpkin seeds, sunflower seeds, bran, cabbage, apples, brewer's yeast, radishes, spinach, almonds, raw oysters, watercress, alfalfa, beef liver, parsley, dried apricots and peaches, molasses, oatmeal, and cooked garlic. These foods, they say, are also helpful for anemics.

Every day walk barefoot through cool dewy grass, run barefoot through chilly white snow, or tread barefoot in a cool bubbly brook (under the cold tap in your tub will do). Why? Because Father Sebastian Kneipp said to, that's why. The famous European water healer made all his patients do it to build up their stamina and health, just as he cured himself of chronic weakness and debilitating diseases by plunging into an icy Bavarian river daily.

The weak who are open-minded may try the following American folk cure from an 1824 healer named J. Monroe: "The milk of a woman is called better than any other for medicinal uses. When this is taken in cases of extreme debility, it should be sucked from the breast of a middle-aged woman of good habits, who lives temperately and uses moderate exercise. The patient should suck about four hours after the woman has taken meals." Ridiculous? Keep in mind that John Wesley's father was "saved" from consumption by sucking thusly some centuries ago.

In our own century, the American Medical Association has finally come around to praising the virtues of mother's milk over man-made formulas for babies; perhaps an AMA endorsement of mother's milk for older debilitated beings is not far off.

WORMS

Intestinal worms have plagued humanity throughout time, but the ancient Greeks, Babylonians, Hindus, Chinese, and Romans knew how to plague the worms: with garlic. So do use it to fight the debilitating little buggers. Modern Canadian nutritionist and garlic enthusiast Paavo Airola suggests that you put a peeled clove of garlic in your shoe if you cannot stand the taste of garlic in your mouth. Then when you walk, the pressure will crush it, releasing its oil to be absorbed through the skin of your foot. This won't solve the problem of how it smells, of course, but for the sake of health you may come to love its distinctive, lingering scent.

Ayurvedic Indian medicine has many remedies for intestinal worms and parasites (and if you've ever been to India you know why). For tapeworm, the Hindus have used pomegranates for centuries. The ancient Greeks prescribed pomegranate seeds for the same ailment, and so did the Arabs. In fact, Prophet Muhammad declared that eating a pomegranate—"purges the system of hate and envy."

Ayurvedic doctors also prescribe unripe papaya juice to expel roundworms: take one tablespoon of the juice of an unripe papaya mixed with one tablespoon of honey and three tablespoons of boiling water, followed two hours later by a dose of castor oil mixed with vinegar. In addition, they say that eating fresh pumpkin seeds, minus their seed coats, will expel all types of intestinal worms and parasites. The Dispensary of the United States, 1894, concurred, describing pumpkin seeds as "one of our most efficient and harmless" expellers of tapeworms.

WOUNDS
AND INFECTIONS

"A wound herb of good respect" is the daisy, so called by Culpeper for its service on the battlefield where it was used in olden days as a healing salve for wounds. Daisies are especially good, according to Culpeper, for wounds in the breast and "ulcers in the secret parts." So please do pick daisies whenever you can. Mix them in a blender or mash into a paste with the back of a spoon and apply externally as needed. Or bathe the wound with a decoction of daisy tea.

Other substances have proved their wound worthiness on the battlefield too. Garlic's antibacterial properties were put to use in World War I by the British army, who applied a mixture of raw garlic juice and water to wounds to prevent infection. In World War II, the Russians used garlic powder on wounds when they were unable to get penicillin.

Honey is another healer. In Shanghai, during World War II, honey was used effectively as a dressing for small wounds and ulcers. It is said to work best when mixed with grease of some kind, particularly butter, which has its own infection-preventing powers. The shamans of central Asia used butter to stop bleeding and to dress wounds, and present-day Tibetans consider butter one of nature's three essences—a "supermedicine"—and the older the better, they say. Contemporary pathologist and medical historian Guido Manjo has discovered that honey and butter combinations are capable of knocking out pathogenic bacteria such as staph and *E. coli.*

The practice of Afro-American healers as well as American Indians and English midwives of the past is to scoop up some cobwebs and place them on cuts to stop bleeding.

Urine has been used for centuries in India for emergency cleansing of external wounds. Healthy urine, say the Indians, makes an excellent bacteria fighter. The ancient Greeks urinated on themselves for this purpose. So do Mexicans, South Americans, and Eskimos.

The Penetientes of New Mexico, who are given to self-flagellation as an act of penitence, favor a wash of cool sage tea to heal their lacerations. Sage's healing powers are numerous and among them is said to be the ability to stop bleeding, soothe wounds, and clean old ulcers and sores. A cooled solution of thyme tea is also highly antiseptic and said to prevent cuts from festering.

For internal infections, give your body an extra supply of infection-fighting iodine

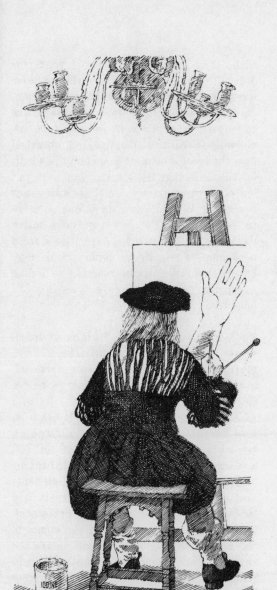

with this suggestion from chiropractor Jairo Rodriguez: Paint the inside of your wrists and forearms with iodine solution. Do it before bedtime so that you don't have to be seen in public with red arms. In the morning it will have disappeared, absorbed into the bloodstream if your body needs it. If the infection is severe, you can put iodine on your arms three times a day, but not more. Whether you do it one or more times a day, do not use it on consecutive days. Rather, use it three days a week for a maximum of two weeks. Some people may have a hypersensitivity reaction to iodine applied to the skin. In rare cases this can be severe.

To help the body heal all kinds of infections, internal and external, take vitamin C throughout the day. Its antibacterial, antiviral action is spectacular; it promotes the production of white blood cells and platelets to help fight infection. It has been said to cure everything from colds to allergies to cancer. Take doses of 500 to 1,000 mg. every four hours for serious infections and diseases, and less for minor ailments and as a daily vitamin supplement. Its only side effect is that, since it is ascorbic acid, it can increase the acidity of the stomach. So people with gastric ulcers should be careful about taking it. To counter the acid reaction, take vitamin C with milk. Rose hips, which contain high amounts of vitamin C, are a natural buffer to the ascorbic acid.

We should all come to love comfrey, a plant known since the Middle Ages as "knitbone," "bruisewort," and "the healing herb." Recently this miraculous plant has been found to contain allantoin, a cell proliferant that helps injured cells heal rapidly. Originally brought from Russia to England, comfrey now grows extensively throughout Europe and North America. While it is not commonly known, owned, or recognized in America, it can easily be grown from rooted clippings or can be procured in most health food stores.

Applied to wounds, bruises, and broken bones comfrey is said to have the power to draw parts together and heal them remarkably fast. The powdered leaf or root, applied to a wound, results in immediate scab formation. In fact, as herbist Joseph Kadams says of it, comfrey "is probably used for more different purposes than any other herb." Its crushed leaves or powder, or poultice or fomentation of same, applied locally are said to cure sores, ulcerated skin, eye injuries, eczema, poison ivy, psoriasis, tumors, itchy anus, headaches, boils, abscesses, milk-swollen breasts, hemorrhoids, gout and arthritic pain, gangrene, burns, and wrinkles caused by malnutrition.

Taken as a tea (a half cupful four times a day) it supposedly helps cure diarrhea, leukorrhea, colds, coughs, digestive complaints, liver problems, bronchial infections, ulcers, malnutrition, and malfunctioning sex drive. Get some today.

APPENDIXES

GENERAL DIRECTIONS FOR TAKING THE CURES

HERBS AND PLANTS

It is preferable to use wild herbs you have picked and prepared yourself. For optimum efficacy, gather herbs in the morning just after the dew has gone, when the plant is in flower and on the second consecutive rainless day. Tie in loose bunches and tenderly hang to dry. Since all this is generally difficult if not impossible to do, buy fresh and dried herbs from herb stores, health food stores, and even supermarkets.

The herbs on your spice rack, while perhaps not the best, still possess natural healing power.

Dried herbs should be stored in dark, dry, airtight containers and should not be subjected to extremes of temperature. They lose strength with passing time, so replace them every couple of years.

The herbs mentioned in this book are safe and gentle when taken as directed. They do not include straightforwardly poisonous or dangerous plants, but allergic reactions are hard to predict and too much of any good thing can be bad, so exercise some caution and common sense. Plants that may prove harmful if taken in excess are listed below.

Unless otherwise noted, take one to three cups of herb tea a day, depending on the severity of the ailment and the potency of the plant. For children, the aged, and the very weak, use approximately half the adult dose.

Prepare herbs (and food) in non-metallic pots, particularly avoiding aluminum utensils because they are said to cause "slow aluminum poisoning" with use, especially when worn or damaged.

Infusion. This is the usual manner of making herb tea. Pour one pint of boiling water over one-half to one ounce of the dried or fresh herb, or one cup of boiling water over one-half to one teaspoon of the plant. Steep, covered, for ten to thirty minutes. Strain and drink.

Decoction. Seeds, roots, fruits, and barks usually have to be boiled for at least ten minutes to extract their healing properties. Use a half-ounce plant part per cup of water. After simmering, cover and let steep another ten minutes or more.

Juice. Squeeze the juice from chopped-up fresh herbs, vegetables, or fruits. An electric juicer makes this a lot easier. Drink soon after making since the fresh juice vitamin power fades rapidly.

Wine. Soak one handful or a few sprigs of the fresh herbs or two tablespoons of the dried variety in a bottle of wine for a few days. For gallon jugs, use one to two ounces of herb.

Poultice. The plant substance is bruised or mashed to a pulp and applied to skin, with moist heat added to it. Mix in a soft adhesive substance like moist flour or bread and milk to make a more easily handled paste. Apply directly or wrap in a cloth and apply cloth pack. Wet with hot water to keep it warm and moist.

Fomentation. Dip a towel or cloth into a strong, hot infusion or decoction. Wring out and apply as hot as possible to the affected area.

WARNING: *The following herbs and spices may be dangerous to your health if abused.* Unless otherwise noted, they have all been classified by the FDA as ''generally recognized as safe.''*

---

* *The best source for cautionary information on herbs is* The Herb Book *by John Lust.*

Camomile. Although it is an extremely mild herb, it can cause dermatitis and a hypersensitivity reaction in patients allergic to ragweed, asters, and other members of the Compositae botanical family. People with such allergies should also avoid *goldenrod* and *marigolds*.

Catnip. Classified by the FDA as an herb of undefined safety, it may cause euphoric or hallucinogenic effects when taken in vast quantities.

Cayenne (capsicum). Lust says excessive consumption may lead to gastroenteritis and kidney damage, but Kloss does not agree. Kloss says cayenne is entirely harmless. To be on the safe side, limit yourself to one cup of the infusion per day, warm, a teaspoon at a time. As a powder, take one to three grains for chronic conditions and three to ten grains for acute conditions.

Comfrey. The FDA considers this an herb of undefined safety.

Ginseng. It has been reported to cause swollen and painful breasts. Some of the Oriental traditions that believe ginseng to be a panacea advise that it not be taken regularly by young people. The FDA classifies the tea as safe but the herb not generally safe as a food additive.

Golden Seal. The FDA classifies it as an herb of undefined safety, and herbalists generally recommend that when it is used internally, it should be taken in weak doses: a quarter teaspoon per cup of hot water.

Licorice. Excessively large amounts can cause sodium and water retention, hypertension, and, in extreme cases, even heart failure and cardiac arrest.

Motherwort. In some individuals it may cause an allergic reaction of dermatitis. The FDA says it is of undefined safety.

Nutmeg. Taken internally in small doses it helps digestion; in large doses it is a narcotic and hallucinogenic. More than two fresh nutmegs consumed at once can be fatal.

Rosemary. Rosemary can be fatal if taken excessively. Drink up to one cup of the tea a day.

Sage. Limit yourself to one cup of the tea a day a tablespoon at a time, since, according to Lust, excessive or extended use can cause symptoms of poisoning. The Chinese and most other herbalists don't agree; they think it can be taken often and is always helpful.

Thyme. Too much thyme tea can overstimulate the thyroid gland. Drink one to two cups a day, a mouthful at a time.

Watercress. In large and regular doses it can damage the kidneys. Do not take it every day or over consistently long periods.

HONEY

Make sure the honey you use is pure, raw honey, unfiltered, uncooked, and unheated (not above 105° F). Most honey found in stores is heated and filtered to make it clearer and easier to package; this destroys enzymes, vitamins, minerals, and trace elements. So do not use that kind for honey cures. Natural honey is usually a little cloudy and crystallizes under cool temperatures.

COLORS

Color therapists say color treatment can be administered in the following manner: Short sunbaths in the nude (sunlight has all colors of the spectrum); absorbing sunlight passed through panes of colored glass (focused onto the ill parts of the body); consume daily a few teaspoons of water that has been set in the sun for a day in a closed, pure colored glass container; massage with oils that have soaked up sun for a month in colored glass containers; use colored clothes, colored surroundings, and colored food; and practice "color breathing"—inhale and visualize colored light, then send it, as breath energy, to the ailing parts of the body.

FASTS

Fasts and mono-diets can be wonderful medicine for all manner of diseases, but long fasts and purification diets should only be undertaken with the guidance of a physician or medical professional. Mono-diets lasting from one to three days are usually quite harmless; however, if you have any special medical problems, it is best to check with a physician before undertaking one.

Always drink plenty of distilled, bottled, or boiled water (tap water will not do) when on a fast or special diet to help flush out accumulated toxins. Also take exercise, baths, and herbal laxatives. And expect to feel a little worse before you feel better: it's the poisons coming out.

GEMS

Gems can be used therapeutically simply by wearing them, preferably close to the skin. Stronger gem medicines can be made and administered orally a few teaspoons a day. Prepare by letting the jewel soak in pure water in a clean glass or porcelain container for a few days. Remove the gem and drink the water. To be effective, gem therapy is supposed to be combined with a healthful and temperate diet.

THE HOLISTIC HEALTH DIET

The cornerstone of the "new" holistic health care mentality is an awareness of nutrition and a reliance on a natural, basically simple diet. Various authorities have claimed that such an eating regimen will not only prevent illness and assuage common complaints but will also cure (in properly modified forms) a host of serious illnesses including heart disease, diabetes, cancer, and multiple sclerosis. Summed up, it amounts to this:

Avoid all refined, processed, canned, and frozen foods, especially all artificial additives and preservatives, all junk food, caffeine, and sugar. Eat less animal products, especially red meat from poor animals that have been raised and slaughtered in unnaturally cruel ways and shot up with hormones, chemical dyes, and God knows what else. Cut down on rich and fat laden foods and whole milk products. Consume mainly whole grains, fresh fruits and vegetables (and their juices), nuts, seeds, beans, sprouted things, honey, and sour milk products like yogurt. Prefer raw foods first and boiled, broiled, and gently sautéed foods in that order. Avoid deep-fried, greasy, and inordinately rich preparations, even if the ingredients are "organic." Always stop eating before you feel really "full." Occasionally go on a short fast or purification diet. And take your organic vitamins every day.

The wise person will adapt this diet to his or her own needs.

SELECTED SOURCES

Airola, Paavo. *The Miracle of Garlic*. Phoenix: Health Plus, 1978.

Anderson, Mary. *Colour Healing*. New York: Samuel Weiser, Inc., 1975.

Bhattcharyya, Benoytosh. *Gem Therapy*. Calcutta: Firma K.L. Mukhopadhyay, 1971.

Bricklin, Mark. *The Practical Encyclopedia of Natural Healing*. Emmaus, Pa.: Rodale Press, 1976.

Buchman, Dian Dincin. *Herbal Medicine*. New York: David McKay, 1979.

Carter, Mildred. *Hand Reflexology*. West Nyack, N.Y.: Parker Publishing Co., 1975.

Clarke, Linda. *A Handbook of Natural Remedies for Common Ailments*. New York: Pocket Books, 1977.

Culpeper's Complete Herbal (17th century). London: Foulsham.

Dastur, J.F. *Everybody's Guide to Ayurvedic Medicine*. Bombay: D.B. Taraporevala Sons, 1972.

Devi, Indra. *Yoga for Americans*. Englewood Cliffs, N.J.: Prentice-Hall, 1959.

Grieve, Mrs. M. *A Modern Herbal*, 2 vols. New York: Dover Publications, 1931, 1971.

Harris, Ben Charles. *The Complete Herbal*. New York: Larchmont Books, 1975.

Hulke, Malcolm, ed. *The Encyclopedia of Alternative Medicine and Self-Help*. New York: Schocken Books, 1979.

Hutchens, Alma R. *Indian Herbalogy of North America*. Ontario: Merco, 1973.

Jarvis, D.C. *Folk Medicine*. New York: Henry Holt and Co., 1958.

Kirschner, H.E. *Nature's Healing Grasses*. Riverside, Calif.: H.C. White Publications, 1960.

Kloss, Jethro. *Back to Eden.* Santa Barbara, Calif.: Woodbridge Press Publishing Co., 1939, 1972.

Kordel, Lelord. *Natural Folk Remedies.* New York: G.P. Putnam's Sons, 1974.

Li Shih-chen. *Chinese Medicinal Herbs* (16th century). Translated by F. Porter Smith and G.A. Stuart. San Francisco: Georgetown Press, 1976.

Lucas, Richard. *Nature's Medicines.* West Nyack, N.Y.: Parker Publishing Co., 1966.

Lust, Benedict. *About Herbs.* London: Thorsons Publishers Ltd., 1961.

Lust, John. *The Herb Book.* New York: Bantam Books, 1974.

Maury, E.A. *Wine Is the Best Medicine.* Kansas City: Sheed, Andrews & McNeel, Inc., 1977.

Mességué, Maurice. *Maurice Mességué's Way to Natural Health and Beauty.* Translated by Clara Winston. New York: Macmillan Publishing Co., Inc., 1974.

Meyer, Clarence. *American Folk Medicine.* New York: Thomas Y. Crowel, 1973.

Namikoshi, Tokujiro. *Shiatsu.* Tokyo: Japan Publications. 1969.

Rechung, Rinpoche. *Tibetan Medicine.* Berkeley: University of California Press, 1973.

Reilly, Dr. Harold J., and Brod, Ruth Hagy. *The Edgar Cayce Handbook for Health Through Drugless Therapy.* New York: Macmillan Publishing Co., Inc., 1975.

Thompson, Robert. *Natural Medicine* (Arabic medicine). New York: McGraw-Hill, 1977.

Thompson, William A.R. *Herbs that Heal.* New York: Charles Scribner's Sons, 1976.

Tisserand, Robert B. *The Art of Aromatherapy.* New York: Inner Traditions International, 1977.

INDEX

Alfalfa, 7, 11, 117, 124
Almonds, 7, 45, 69–70, 124
Aloe vera plant, 26
Anise, 23, 37, 57, 100, 107
Apples, 6, 87, 95, 96, 104, 117, 124
Apricots, 7, 124
Asparagus, 87, 106

Baking soda,54, 83, 113, 117
Bananas, 44–45
Basil, 51, 74, 78, 94, 107
Bathing, 95, 113
Beets, 42, 44
Blueberries, 30, 44, 118
Bran, 7, 41, 77, 86–87, 124
Bread, 24, 103, 104
Brewer's yeast, 7, 124
Butter, 127–28

Cabbage, 27, 64, 100, 105, 124
Camomile, 59, 74, 78, 87, 94, 95, 136
Caraway, 20, 57, 107
Carrots, 24, 45, 53, 87, 95, 105
Catnip, 30, 51–52, 100, 136
Celery, 9–10, 27, 95, 96, 106
Chervil, 87, 91
Chicken soup, 35–37, 106
Chick-peas, 83
Cinnamon, 32, 37, 75, 107
Clove, 37, 60, 91, 94, 118
Coffee, 18, 20, 63
Comfrey, 131, 136

Corn silk, 79, 81
Cornstarch, 113
Cottonseed oil, 89
Cranberry juice, 82
Cream, sour, 114–15
Cucumber, 23, 28, 50, 114

Daisy, 100, 127
Dandelions, 9, 11, 30, 68, 85–86, 122
Date, 8, 60
Decoction, 135
Diamonds, 108
Dill, 57, 70

Egg(s), 24, 92
Emeralds, 85
Emotions, negative, 6, 77, 99
Eucalyptus, 55–56, 110
Exercises
  barefoot walking, 124–25
  breathing, 27, 30, 71, 98
  "corpse pose," 97
  half-headstand, 91–92
  for hemorrhoids (Cayce's cure), 69
  mantric sound, 71
  massage, 27, 32, 59–60, 65–66, 78, 89, 110
  meditation, 71–72
  neti (yoga), 110
  "rabbit" pose, 57–58
  running-in-place, 66
  shoulder stand, 102–103
  vision (palming), 48, 50
  "wind-removing" yoga pose, 57

Fasts, 138–39
Fennel, 27, 47, 50–51, 57, 91, 107
Fenugreek, 107, 109
Flower remedies, 99, 121
Fomentation, 135

Garlic, 7, 16, 18, 23, 29, 32–33, 37–38, 46, 72,
    86, 105, 106, 109, 124, 125–26, 127
Geranium, 117–18
Ginger, 30, 32, 34, 37, 51, 60, 61, 75, 84, 91,
    93, 106, 107
Ginseng, 2–3, 4, 106, 124, 136
Golden seal, 30, 109, 115–16, 118, 136
Grapes, 38–40, 83, 87

Herbs, vii–viii, x–xii, 8, 133–35
Holistic health diet, vii–ix, x, 139–40
Honey, 11, 16, 22, 23, 41, 45–46, 61, 63, 64, 68,
    78, 104, 106, 107, 114, 115, 119, 127–28,
    137–38
Horseradish, 110–11

Infusion, 134
Iodine solution, 103, 129–30
Ivy, 28, 65

Jasmine, 95, 107–108

Kidney beans, 81, 88

Lavender, 22, 27, 95–96
Lemon, 11, 16–17, 41, 42, 45, 84, 86, 111, 115
Lettuce, 4, 100
Licorice, 3–4, 17–18, 106–107, 119, 137

Magnolia bark, 54–55
Marigold, 30, 121
Marijuana, 44, 48, 93
Marjoram, 77, 78, 87, 94
Milk, 37, 39, 42, 70, 77–78, 81–82, 106, 125
Mint, 20, 65, 75, 87, 93, 105
Molasses, 7, 53, 124
Moonstone, 103, 104
Mullein, 12, 15, 42, 116

Nature cures ("naturopathy"), ix–x
Nutmeg, 54, 107, 114, 137

Oatmeal, 7, 124
Oats, 88–89
Olive oil, 41, 46, 61, 64
Onions, 16, 27, 33, 46, 50, 55, 60–61, 66–67, 78,
    82, 105–106, 122
Orange juice, 52, 56, 70, 95
Oregano, 78, 94
Oysters, 7, 88, 106, 124

Papayas, 42, 75–76, 114, 116, 126
Parsley, 7, 11, 22, 27, 47, 59, 79, 87, 124
Peaches, 7, 93, 106, 124
Pepper, 18, 107
Peppermint, 30, 45, 65, 67–68, 100, 110
Plants, 133–35
Pomegranates, 34–35, 126
Potato, 12, 26, 35, 105, 122
Pumpkin, 7, 82, 88, 124, 126

Radish, 7, 87, 122, 124
Raisins, 84
Ram testicle (rooster kidney) soup, 105
Raspberry leaf, 52
Red pepper (cayenne), 30, 35, 56, 63, 120–21
Rosemary, 5–6, 13, 20, 27, 32, 51, 65, 87, 89–90,
    106, 107, 122, 137
Roses, 13, 30, 44, 68, 87, 95, 107, 108
Rubies, 9, 34

Saffron, 7, 30, 54, 88
Sage, 33, 44, 51, 53, 54, 73–74, 87, 90–91, 94,
    96, 100, 118, 122, 128, 137

Salt, 63, 103, 114, 118, 124
Sandalwood oil, 95, 107
Seaweed, 103, 124
Sesame, 29, 70, 107
Sexual habits, 82–83, 94–95
Sleeping bag cure, 12–13
Soybeans, 29
Spinach, 7, 87, 95, 124
Strawberries, 11, 28, 45, 83, 87, 114, 116, 117
Sunflower, 7, 18, 124

Tangerine tea, 23
Teas
    black, 108
    Earl Grey, 56
    herbal, 52, 57
    jackrabbit turd, 55
Therapies
    acupressure, 65, 78
    acupuncture, xiii, 63
    aromatherapy, xiii, 27
    Ayurvedic, 11, 44–45, 46, 84, 88, 126
    black folk medicine, 29
    color, xiii, 4–5, 34, 76, 95, 138
    energy cures, xii–xiii
    finger pressure, 101–102, 108
    gem, xiii, 9, 85, 103–104, 108, 139
    mind cures, xiii–xiv
    reflexology, xiii, 19–20, 27, 60, 63, 110
    yoga, xiii, 6–7, 18–19, 71, 78–79, 98
Thyme, 8, 30, 33, 51, 63, 74, 94, 100, 107,
    113, 122, 128, 137
Toadstool, 116
Tonic, herbal, 84–85
Topaz, 103, 104

Urine, 46, 111–13, 128

Vinegar, 11, 54, 105, 116
Violets, 30, 118
Vitamins
    A, 24, 114
    B (niacinamide), 30, 61, 78, 96–97, 114
    B_6 (pyridoxine), 17, 84, 108, 109, 114
    C, 34, 68, 84, 118, 130
    E, 61, 67, 84, 108, 109, 114, 121, 122

Water, 10, 11–12, 26, 27, 32, 41, 45, 58, 72–73,
    101, 104, 107, 110, 113, 114, 116, 118, 119
Watercress, 7, 11, 87, 95, 124, 137
Wine, 7, 8–9, 18, 28–29, 38, 67, 74, 114, 135

Yams, 4, 53
Yellow in color therapy, 76
Yogurt, 11, 26, 38, 39, 42, 53, 114